Religious Responses to HIV and AIDS

Drawing on a wide range of methodologies, this book documents a diverse portfolio of religious responses to HIV and AIDS on the local and global levels at sites from sub-Saharan Africa to New York City. The volume goes beyond the psychology of religion, which is often based on how religion is used to cope with illness. It seeks to examine the role of religious institutions and cultures as key players in civil society, and to examine not only psychological factors, but social, cultural, economic and political dimensions of religious responses to the AIDS epidemic. Religious movements have, at times, provided powerful forces for community mobilisation in response to the social vulnerability, economic exclusion and health problems associated with HIV. In other contexts, religious cultures have reproduced values and practices that have seriously impeded more effective approaches to mitigate the epidemic. By highlighting these complex and sometimes contradictory social processes, this book provides new insights into the potential for religious institutions to address the HIV epidemic more effectively. More broadly, it demonstrates how research on religion can inform public health, illustrating how civil society organisations shape opportunities for health promotion: a crucial and new area of global public health research.

This book was originally published as a special issue of *Global Public Health*.

Miguel Muñoz-Laboy is an Associate Professor at Temple University, USA, and a public health and social work researcher whose work focuses on the intersections of social and cultural factors as determinants of HIV risk.

Jonathan Garcia is an Associate Research Scientist at Columbia University, USA, and a political anthropologist with extensive field research focused on HIV and AIDS and community mobilisation in Brazil and the United States.

Joyce Moon-Howard is an Assistant Professor of Clinical Sociomedical Sciences at Columbia University, USA, and a specialist in community-involved public health research primarily among minority communities with a long-standing research and programmatic interest in religious responses to HIV and AIDS domestically and internationally.

Patrick A. Wilson is an Associate Professor of Sociomedical Sciences at Columbia University, USA, and a community psychologist with more than a decade of experience examining the intersecting roles that psychological factors and socio-contextual factors (i.e., discrimination and stigma, religion) play in explaining HIV risk and protective behaviours among racial/ethnic and sexual minority populations.

Richard Parker is a Professor of Sociomedical Sciences and Anthropology at Columbia University, USA, and is one of the pioneer scholars in examining the structural factors and political economy of the global HIV/AIDS epidemic.

Religious Responses to HIV and AIDS

Edited by
Miguel Muñoz-Laboy, Jonathan Garcia, Joyce Moon-Howard, Patrick A. Wilson, and Richard Parker

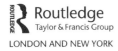
LONDON AND NEW YORK

First published 2015
by Routledge
2 Park Square, Milton Park, Abingdon, Oxon, OX14 4RN, UK

and by Routledge
711 Third Avenue, New York, NY 10017, USA

Routledge is an imprint of the Taylor & Francis Group, an informa business

British Library Cataloguing in Publication Data
A catalogue record for this book is available from the British Library

ISBN13: 978-1-138-79367-5

Typeset in Times New Roman
by Taylor & Francis Books

Publisher's Note
The publisher accepts responsibility for any inconsistencies that may have arisen during the conversion of this book from journal articles to book chapters, namely the possible inclusion of journal terminology.

Disclaimer
Every effort has been made to contact copyright holders for their permission to reprint material in this book. The publishers would be grateful to hear from any copyright holder who is not here acknowledged and will undertake to rectify any errors or omissions in future editions of this book.

Contents

Citation Information   vii

1. Introduction: Religious responses to HIV and AIDS: Understanding
   the role of religious cultures and institutions in confronting the epidemic
   Miguel Muñoz-Laboy, Jonathan Garcia, Joyce Moon-Howard,
   Patrick A. Wilson and Richard Parker   1

2. AIDS, religious enthusiasm and spiritual insecurity in Africa
   Adam Ashforth   6

3. Fighting down the scourge, building up the church: Organisational
   constraints in religious involvement with HIV/AIDS in Mozambique
   Victor Agadjanian and Cecilia Menjívar   22

4. Pentecostalism and AIDS treatment in Mozambique: Creating new
   approaches to HIV prevention through anti-retroviral therapy
   James Pfeiffer   37

5. Free love: A case study of church-run home-based caregivers in a high
   vulnerability setting
   Robin Root and Arnau van Wyngaard   48

6. Conflicts between conservative Christian institutions and secular groups
   in sub-Saharan Africa: Ideological discourses on sexualities, reproduction
   and HIV/AIDS
   Joanne E. Mantell, Jacqueline Correale, Jessica Adams-Skinner and
   Zena A. Stein   66

7. Civic/sanctuary orientation and HIV involvement among Chinese
   immigrant religious institutions in New York City
   John J. Chin, Min Ying Li, Ezer Kang, Elana Behar and
   Po Chun Chen   84

8. Ideologies of Black churches in New York City and the public health
   crisis of HIV among Black men who have sex with men
   Patrick A. Wilson, Natalie M. Wittlin, Miguel Muñoz-Laboy and
   Richard Parker   101

CONTENTS

9. Vulnerable salvation: Evangelical Protestant leaders and institutions, drug use and HIV and AIDS in the urban periphery of Rio de Janeiro
Jonathan Garcia, Miguel Muñoz-Laboy and Richard Parker   117

10. Blood, sweat and semen: The economy of *axé* and the response of Afro-Brazilian religions to HIV and AIDS in Recife
Luis Felipe Rios, Cinthia Oliveira, Jonathan Garcia, Miguel Muñoz-Laboy, Laura Murray and Richard Parker   131

11. A time for dogma, a time for the Bible, a time for condoms: Building a Catholic theology of prevention in the face of public health policies at Casa Fonte Colombo in Porto Alegre, Brazil
Fernando Seffner, Jonathan Garcia, Miguel Muñoz-Laboy and Richard Parker   145

Index   159

Citation Information

The chapters in this book were originally published in *Global Public Health*, volume 6, issue S2 (October 2011). When citing this material, please use the original page numbering for each article, as follows:

Chapter 1
Introduction: Religious responses to HIV and AIDS: Understanding the role of religious cultures and institutions in confronting the epidemic
Miguel Muñoz-Laboy, Jonathan Garcia, Joyce Moon-Howard, Patrick A. Wilson and Richard Parker
Global Public Health, volume 6, issue S2 (October 2011) pp. S127-S131

Chapter 2
AIDS, religious enthusiasm and spiritual insecurity in Africa
Adam Ashforth
Global Public Health, volume 6, issue S2 (October 2011) pp. S132-S147

Chapter 3
Fighting down the scourge, building up the church: Organisational constraints in religious involvement with HIV/AIDS in Mozambique
Victor Agadjanian and Cecilia Menjívar
Global Public Health, volume 6, issue S2 (October 2011) pp. S148-S162

Chapter 4
Pentecostalism and AIDS treatment in Mozambique: Creating new approaches to HIV prevention through anti-retroviral therapy
James Pfeiffer
Global Public Health, volume 6, issue S2 (October 2011) pp. S163-S173

Chapter 5
Free love: A case study of church-run home-based caregivers in a high vulnerability setting
Robin Root and Arnau van Wyngaard
Global Public Health, volume 6, issue S2 (October 2011) pp. S174-S191

Chapter 6

Conflicts between conservative Christian institutions and secular groups in sub-Saharan Africa: Ideological discourses on sexualities, reproduction and HIV/AIDS
Joanne E. Mantell, Jacqueline Correale, Jessica Adams-Skinner and Zena A. Stein
Global Public Health, volume 6, issue S2 (October 2011) pp. S192-S209

Chapter 7

Civic/sanctuary orientation and HIV involvement among Chinese immigrant religious institutions in New York City
John J. Chin, Min Ying Li, Ezer Kang, Elana Behar and Po Chun Chen
Global Public Health, volume 6, issue S2 (October 2011) pp. S210-S226

Chapter 8

Ideologies of Black churches in New York City and the public health crisis of HIV among Black men who have sex with men
Patrick A. Wilson, Natalie M. Wittlin, Miguel Muñoz-Laboy and Richard Parker
Global Public Health, volume 6, issue S2 (October 2011) pp. S227-S242

Chapter 9

Vulnerable salvation: Evangelical Protestant leaders and institutions, drug use and HIV and AIDS in the urban periphery of Rio de Janeiro
Jonathan Garcia, Miguel Muñoz-Laboy and Richard Parker
Global Public Health, volume 6, issue S2 (October 2011) pp. S243-S256

Chapter 10

Blood, sweat and semen: The economy of axé *and the response of Afro-Brazilian religions to HIV and AIDS in Recife*
Luis Felipe Rios, Cinthia Oliveira, Jonathan Garcia, Miguel Muñoz-Laboy, Laura Murray and Richard Parker
Global Public Health, volume 6, issue S2 (October 2011) pp. S257-S270

Chapter 11

A time for dogma, a time for the Bible, a time for condoms: Building a Catholic theology of prevention in the face of public health policies at Casa Fonte Colombo in Porto Alegre, Brazil
Fernando Seffner, Jonathan Garcia, Miguel Muñoz-Laboy and Richard Parker
Global Public Health, volume 6, issue S2 (October 2011) pp. S271-S283

INTRODUCTION

Religious responses to HIV and AIDS: Understanding the role of religious cultures and institutions in confronting the epidemic

Miguel Muñoz-Laboy[a], Jonathan Garcia[b], Joyce Moon-Howard[a], Patrick A. Wilson[a] and Richard Parker[a]

[a]Department of Sociomedical Sciences, Mailman School of Public Health, Columbia University, New York, NY, USA; [b]Center for Interdisciplinary Research on AIDS, Yale School of Public Health, Yale University, New Haven, CT, USA

Since the very beginning of the HIV epidemic, few social institutions have been as important as religion in shaping the ways in which individuals, communities and societies have responded to HIV and AIDS. In societies around the world, what are sometimes described as religious belief systems or religious cultures have been fundamental to the interpretation of AIDS – to the ways in which a newly emerging infectious disease was incorporated into existing understandings of the world. Over the course of more than three decades now, religious meaning systems have mediated the attitudes and policies related to the epidemic and public health programmes, and religious organisations have been central to the response to HIV and AIDS in countries and cultures around the world (Lagarde *et al.* 2000, Agadjanian 2005, Global Health Council 2005, McGirk 2008, Garcia *et al.* 2009, Akintola 2010, Murray *et al.* 2011, Trinitapoli 2011). This impact has been profoundly complex and often contradictory.

At the same time, religious organisations play a key role globally in providing front-line access to primary and terminal care, advocating for health and social welfare resources and influencing public health and social policies (Sanders 1997, Chatter 2000, DeHaven *et al.* 2004, Pargament *et al.* 2004). This has been especially visible in relation to the global HIV epidemic, and has expanded significantly over the past decade as part of the global scale-up of HIV programmes (Shelp and Sunderland 1992, Global Health Council 2005). Agencies such as the World Health Organisation, Joint United Nations Programme on HIV/AIDS (UNAIDS), the Global Fund to Fight AIDS, Tuberculosis and Malaria, and the US President's Emergency Plan for AIDS Relief (PEPFAR) programme have all called for increased involvement of and partnerships with community-based organisations (CBOs) and faith-based organisations (FBOs) as part of the expanded global response to AIDS (Global Health Council 2005, United Nations Population Fund [UNFPA] 2008a, 2008b, UNAIDS 2009). With the assistance of international donor agencies, millions of dollars are now spent annually to support interventions by religious institutions and FBOs for HIV prevention and treatment in the developing world, and the WHO estimates that at least one in five organisations involved in HIV/AIDS programming is now faith-based (WHO 2004, Agadjanian 2005, Global Health Council 2005, Agadjanian and Sen 2007, Akintola 2010). However, concerns have been raised that this growing emphasis on the role of FBOs has been based more on ideological convictions than on empirical evidence about their effectiveness. A scientific understanding of the role of FBOs in responding to the HIV epidemic remains almost non-existent. The few assessments that exist all point to the urgent need for further empirical investigation of the activities of FBOs and more rigorous evaluation of the interventions they deliver in response to HIV and AIDS (Global Health Council 2005).

One of the key reasons for the lack of meaningful research on the many complex dimensions of the religious response to HIV and AIDS has been the fact that much of the research examining religion in relation to population health needs has tended to focus primarily on identifying the effects of what have been described as religious beliefs on individual health behaviour and outcomes (Woods and Ironson 1999, Duan et al. 2000), without looking critically at religion as a social force that shapes social, cultural, and institutional responses to health conditions and health disparities (Remle and Koenig 2001, Simoni and Ortiz 2003, Prado et al. 2004). In the study of religious responses to the epidemic, as in HIV and AIDS research more broadly, there is thus an urgent need to move towards a broader focus aimed at understanding not just individual health behaviours and outcomes, but the broader social and cultural settings within which behaviour takes place – and the broader social and political forces that shape it.

Religious responses to HIV and AIDS provide an ideal focus from which to examine institutional religious involvement in health precisely because of the controversies that the AIDS epidemic has brought to the forefront of social, scientific and policy debates (Muñoz-Laboy et al. 2011). In distinct contexts throughout sub-Saharan Africa, Asia, Latin America and North America researchers have increasingly shown how social inequality, combined with rising HIV incidence rates and the presence of international organisations, has affected the way in which religious cultures and institutions have responded to the epidemic, often creating tension between traditional beliefs and 'new' religious cultures that have entered countries along with NGOs and donor agencies (Pfeiffer 2002, 2004, 2005, Agadjanian 2005, Swidler 2009, Paiva et al. 2010, Garcia and Parker 2011, Murray et al. 2011).

The articles that have been included in this Special Supplement of *Global Public Health* provide important examples of some of the kinds of research that we think is so urgently needed in order to more fully understand the complexity of religious traditions and FBOs as they have responded to the HIV/AIDS epidemic both globally and locally. While the work that is presented in these articles is highly diverse, it is nonetheless characterised by a focus on religious cultures and institutions. The articles that are included here draw heavily on a long history of research in fields such as the sociology and anthropology of religion, and in the multidisciplinary field of the comparative study of religions (Bellah 1970, Calhoun 1991, Dillon 2003). They approach the study of religion as a social and cultural system (Bellah 1970, Geertz 1973, Lessa 1979, Lambek 2002). This approach focuses on the ways in which these systems are articulated through the organisational structures of different religious denominations (and different currents of thought within specific denominations), in seeking not only to shape the behaviour of religious believers, but also to influence and impact the secular world more broadly (Bellah 1970). It thus helps us to understand the ways in which religious organisations can become among the most important institutional actors in civil society in relation to a wide range of social and political issues (Bellah 1970, Geertz 1973, Calhoun 1991). While this approach has seldom been utilised in the study of public health issues, it nonetheless suggests a number of ways in which religious organisations can have a major impact in shaping vulnerability and prevention as well as treatment and care – an impact that has still been only minimally investigated in the research literature on HIV and AIDS.

The articles focus on systems of cultural meaning and social and structural factors that both shape the epidemic and condition the responses that different communities and societies are able to offer in relation to it, and the understanding of religion as a social and cultural system. This is articulated through organisational structures that constitute among the most important institutional actors in civil society. These articles also highlight the extent to which religious organisations must be understood as key institutional actors within social movements that have emerged as part of the broader social response to the epidemic. One of the major outcomes of the comparative study of religious systems as they impact social action has been a growing sense that religions must themselves be understood as social movements (often highly conservative, but sometimes very progressive as well) precisely because they often explicitly seek to take steps aimed at transforming the world around them, frequently in the name of poor, marginalised and excluded population groups (Yarnold 1991, Scheie and Markham 1994, Wittberg 1994, Lucas and Robbins 2004).

The articles in this Special Supplement document the complex ways in which diverse religious traditions in different societies have contributed to the broader social response to HIV and AIDS, as well as they ways in which they have shaped the more localised responses of their followers. Religious meaning systems, practices and institutions have been central to the articulation of projects for social change of diverse types in response to HIV and AIDS. Sometimes, religious cultures have reproduced values and practices that have seriously impeded more effective approaches to mitigate the epidemic. At other times, religious movements have provided among the most powerful forces for the mobilisation of individuals and communities in response to the social vulnerability, economic exclusion and public health risk associated with HIV. By highlighting these complex and sometimes contradictory social processes, the analyses developed in this Special Supplement provide new insights not only into the relationship between religion and the HIV epidemic, but between religion and global public health more broadly, thus helping to open up a crucial new area of global public health research.

Acknowledgements

The articles that have been included in this Special Supplement were all originally prepared for the conference 'Religious Responses to HIV and AIDS' that was organised with support from a grant (#1 R13 HD066966-01) from the US Eunice Kennedy Shriver National Institute of Child Health and Human Development (NICHD). Additional support for the conference, and for the publication of this Special Supplement, has been provided by the Center for the Study of Culture, Politics and Health, Department of Sociomedical Sciences, Mailman School of Public Health at Columbia University. The views expressed here are solely those of the authors and do not reflect the opinions of any of the institutions that have provided support for this publication.

References

Agadjanian, V., 2005. Gender, religious involvement, and HIV/AIDS prevention in Mozambique. *Social Science and Medicine*, 61 (7), 1529–1539.

Agadjanian, V. and Sen, S., 2007. Promises and challenges of faith-based AIDS care and support in Mozambique. *American Journal of Public Health*, 97 (2), 362–366.

Akintola, O., 2010. Perceptions of rewards among volunteer caregivers of people living with AIDS working in faith-based organizations in South Africa: a qualitative study. *Journal of the International AIDS Society*, 13 (22), 1–10.

Bellah, R.N., 1970. *Beyond belief: essays on religion in a post-traditional world*. New York: Harper & Row.

Calhoun, C.J., 1991. *Comparative social research: religious institutions*. Greenwich, CT: JAI Press.

Chatter, L., 2000. Religion and health: public health research and practice. *Annual Review of Public Health*, 21, 335–367.

DeHaven, M.J., Hunter, I.B., Wilder, L., Walton, J.W., and Berry, J., 2004. Health programs in faith-based organizations: are they effective? *American Journal of Public Health*, 94 (6), 1030–1036.

Dillon, M., 2003. *Handbook of the sociology of religion*. Cambridge: Cambridge University Press.

Duan, N., Fox, S.A., Derose, K.P., and Carson, S., 2000. Maintaining mammography adherence through telephone counseling in a church based trial. *American Journal of Public Health*, 90 (9), 1468–1471.

Garcia, J., Muñoz-Laboy, M., de Almeida, V., and Parker, R., 2009. Local impacts of religious discourses on rights to express same-sex desires in peri-urban Rio de Janeiro. *Sexuality Research and Social Policy*, 6 (3), 44–60.

Garcia, J. and Parker, R., 2011. Resource mobilization for health advocacy: Afro-Brazilian religious organizations and HIV prevention and control. *Social Science and Medicine*, 72 (12), 1930–1938.

Geertz, C., 1973. Religion as a cultural system. *In: The interpretation of cultures*. New York: Basic Books, 87–125.

Global Health Council, 2005. *Faith in action: examining the role of faith-based organizations in addressing HIV/AIDS* [online]. Available from: http://www.globalhealth.org/view_top.php3? id=448 [Accessed 12 June 2010].

Lagarde, E., Enel, C., Seck, K., Gueye-Ndiaye, A., Piau, J., Pison, G., Delaunay, V., Ndoye, I., and Mboup, S., 2000. Religion and protective behaviours towards AIDS in rural Senegal. *AIDS*, 14 (13), 2027–2033.

Lambek, M., 2002. *A reader in the anthropology of religion*. Malden, MA: Blackwell.

Lessa, W.A., 1979. *Reader in comparative religion: an anthropological approach*. 4th ed. New York: Harper & Row.

Lucas, P.C. and Robbins, T., 2004. *New religious movements in the 21st century: legal, political and social challenges in global perspective*. New York: Routledge.

McGirk, J., 2008. Religious leaders key in the Middle East's HIV/AIDS fight. *Lancet*, 372 (9635), 279–280.

Muñoz-Laboy, M., Murray, L.R., Wittlin, N., Garcia, J., Terto, V., and Parker, R., 2011. Beyond faith-based organizations: using comparative institutional ethnography to understand religious responses to HIV and AIDS in Brazil. *American Journal of Public Health*, 1 (6), 972–978.

Murray, L., Garcia, J., Muñoz-Laboy, M., and Parker, R., 2011. Strange bedfellows: the Catholic Church and Brazilian National AIDS Program in the response to AIDS in Brazil. *Social Science and Medicine*, 72 (6), 945–952.

Paiva, V., Garcia, J., Rios, L.F., Santos, A., Terto, V., and Muñoz-Laboy, M., 2010. Religious communities and HIV prevention: an intervention study using a human rights-based approach. *Global Public Health*, 5 (3), 284–290.

Pargament, K.I., McCarthy, S., Shah, P., Ano, G., Tarakeshwar, N., Wachholtz, A., Sirrine, N., Vasconcelles, E., Murray-Swank, N., Locher, A., and Duggan, J., 2004. Religion and HIV: a review of the literature and clinical implications. *Southern Medical Journal*, 97 (12), 1201–1209.

Pfeiffer, J., 2002. African independent churches in Mozambique: healing the afflictions of inequality. *Medical Anthropology Quarterly*, 16 (2), 176–199.

Pfeiffer, J., 2004. Condom social marketing, Pentecostalism, and structural adjustment in Mozambique: a clash of AIDS prevention messages. *Medical Anthropology Quarterly*, 18 (1), 77–103.

Pfeiffer, J., 2005. Commodity fetichismo, the Holy Spirit, and the turn to Pentecostal and African Independent Churches in Central Mozambique. *Culture, Medicine and Psychiatry*, 29 (3), 255–283.

Prado, G., Feaster, D., Schwartz, S., Pratt, I., Smith, L., and Szapocznik, J., 2004. Religious involvement, coping, social support, and psychological distress in HIV-seropositive African American mothers. *AIDS and Behavior*, 8 (3), 221–235.

Remle, R.C. and Koenig, H.G., 2001. Religion and health in HIV/AIDS communities. *In*: T.G. Plante and A.C. Sherman, eds. *Faith and health: psychological perspectives*. New York: Guilford Press, 195–212.

Sanders, E.C., 1997. New insights and interventions: churches uniting to reach the African American community with health information. *Journal of Health Care for the Poor and Underserved*, 8 (3), 373–375.

Scheie, D.M. and Markham, J., 1994. *Better together: religious institutions as partners in community-based development*. Minneapolis, MN: Rainbow Research.

Shelp, E.E. and Sunderland, R.H., 1992. *AIDS and the Church*. Louisville, KY: Westminster/John Knox Press.

Simoni, J. and Ortiz, M., 2003. Mediational models of spirituality and depressive symptomatology among HIV-positive Puerto Rican women. *Cultural Diversity and Ethnic Minority Psychology*, 9 (1), 3–15.

Swidler, A., 2009. Responding to AIDS in sub-Saharan Africa. *In*: P. Hall and M. Lamont, eds. *Successful societies: institutions, cultural repertoires and population health*. Cambridge: Cambridge University Press, 128–150.

Trinitapoli, J., 2011. The AIDS-related activities of religious leaders in Malawi. *Global Public Health*, 6 (1), 41–55.

UNAIDS, 2009. *Partnership with faith-based organizations: UNAIDS strategic framework* [online]. Available from: http://data.unaids.org/pub/BaseDocument/2009/jc1786partnershipwithfaithbasedorganizations_en.pdf [Accessed 10 June 2010].

UNFPA, 2008a. *Proceedings report: United Nations inter-agency consultation on engagement with faith-based organizations* [online]. Available from: http://www.unfpa.org/webdav/site/global/shared/documents/publications/2008/proceedings_fbo.pdf [Accessed 12 June 2010].

UNFPA, 2008b. *Culture matters: a legacy from engaging faith-based organizations* [online]. Available from: http://www.unfpa.org/webdav/site/global/shared/documents/publications/2008/Culture_Matter_II.pdf [Accessed 12 June 2010].

Wittberg, P., 1994. *The rise and decline of Catholic religious orders: a social movement perspective*. Albany: State University of New York Press.

Woods, T.E. and Ironson, G.H., 1999. Religion and spirituality in the face of illness: how cancer, cardiac, and HIV patients describe their spirituality/religiosity. *Journal of Health Psychology*, 4 (3), 393–412.

World Health Organization [WHO], 2004. *World health report 2004: changing history* [online]. Available from: http://www.who.int/whr/2004/en/report04_en.pdf [Accessed 14 February 2011].

Yarnold, B., 1991. *The role of religious organization in social movements*. New York: Praeger.

AIDS, religious enthusiasm and spiritual insecurity in Africa

Adam Ashforth

Department of Afroamerican and African Studies, University of Michigan, Ann Arbor, MI, USA

The connection between the AIDS epidemic and the efflorescence of religious 'enthusiasm' (construed in both classical and contemporary senses) in Africa in recent decades is best understood, this paper argues, by reference to a concept of 'spiritual insecurity'. The article offers a general description of the condition of spiritual insecurity and argues that it is best studied within a relational realist paradigm. The article presents a critique of the concept of 'belief' as commonly used in the social science of religion, arguing instead for an opening of the study of social relations to include the universe of relations within which people experience the world, including their relations with entities such as spiritual beings that might otherwise be considered virtual.

Introduction: AIDS, religious enthusiasm and a miracle cure in Tanzania

In August 2010, in the remote northern Tanzanian village of Samunge in Loliondo, 325 km north of the nearest town, Arusha, God spoke to a 75-year-old retired pastor of the Evangelical Lutheran Church, Mr. Anbilikile Mwasapila, and gave him the recipe for a miraculous medicine. By boiling the bark of the 'mugagira' tree and dispensing it to patients one cup at a time, God would cure people of AIDS, cancer, diabetes, high blood pressure, asthma, and anything else that ailed them (Guardian-on-Sunday-Team 2011).

Word spread quickly of the 'wonders' being performed at Loliondo. By early 2011, stories were appearing in newspapers and on radio and television across East Africa. Tens of thousands of people made the difficult journey to Loliondo for a cup of Mr. Mwasapila's medicine. By March, traffic to the village was backed up for 15 km. Thousands claimed to have been cured, including Members of Parliament and Judges who 'testified' to the medicine's efficacy. Others, not yet ill, trekked to Mr. Mwasapila's bucket to gain protection from future harm. Gravely ill patients were dying on the road to the cure. (Tour operators recommend that people unable to handle the 6-hour journey by road from Arusha take a helicopter. See www. loliondotravels.com.) Health Ministers from Kenya and Tanzania warned the public against trusting untested medicines but were constrained in attempting to regulate Mr. Mwasapila's enterprise by his phenomenal popularity. Doctors in Arusha saw the wards of the hospital emptying of patients (NTV Kenya 2011). Mr. Mwasapila was modest in the price he charged for his miracle drink, only 500 Tanzanian

Shillings (about 30 cents), but was not circumspect in his claims: the brew could cure AIDS, cancer, diabetes, high blood pressure, asthma. Everything. God is great.

Mr. Mwasapila's miracle cure is but one of thousands of similar phenomena in recent decades in Africa, notable only for the scale of his operations and the publicity he has received. In the mid-1990s, for example, a Malawian villager treated more than a million people with his 'cure' for AIDS (Probst 1999, Schoffeleers 1999, Doran 2007). Across the continent, hundreds of thousands (if not millions) of healers are brewing their decoctions daily, usually with recipes inspired by communication with spiritual beings of one kind or another. A similar number work directly with God, Jesus, the Holy Ghost, Allah, ancestors, or other invisible beings spoken of in doctrines of religion to cure illness, restore good relations in families and communities, bring wealth and good fortune, cast out demons, protect against witchcraft and sorcery, and much, much, more.

In this article I argue that the key to understanding phenomena such as the Loliondo miracle cure and the connection between AIDS and religious enthusiasm more generally, is the concept of 'spiritual insecurity' referring to the sense of danger, doubt, and fear arising from efforts to manage relations with invisible forces. I present the outline of a framework for thinking about religious culture and AIDS in contemporary Africa in terms of a paradigm of security, which incorporates a broad field of power relations in the scope of analysis. This framework, I argue, allows us to move beyond approaches that focus on questions of belief in relation to healing and religion in order to analyse the broad range of forces that people experience as shaping their lives in all dimensions.[1]

So, how should we interpret something like the Loliondo wonder?

Religious enthusiasm: a relational realist approach

The most appropriate term for describing events at Loliondo, it seems to me, is 'religious enthusiasm'. In the original Greek, from whence it derives, the term enthusiasm means possessed by a god (en/theos). In the seventeenth and eighteenth centuries, in England, it was used to disparage Protestant religious movements promising a direct connection with the Almighty (Knox 1950). David Hume (1963 [1742–1754]), for example, wrote an essay denouncing enthusiasm as a corrupted form of religion, an equivalent, if opposite, delusion to priest-ridden superstition. In the twentieth century, the term has come to signify a positive, energetic, embrace of something (Tucker 1972). I use enthusiasm here in all these senses. The term is particularly apposite, given the long history and contemporary traditions of spirit possession in Africa and the centrality of relations with invisible beings in African practices of healing (Behrend and Luig 1999, Kalu 2009). Enthusiasm, it should be noted, is by no means exclusive to Christians (PewForum 2010, Manglos and Trinitapoli 2011). Since Christianity predominates in the regions of Africa most affected by generalised AIDS epidemics, however, I shall concentrate on Christianity here.

Mr. Mwasapila claims to have communicated directly with God in the making of his medicine. His medicine, which has to be dispensed directly from his hand – hence the need for people to trek out to his village rather have it shipped to town in tankers – substantiates a relationship with God mediated by Mr. Mwasapila. God has chosen this substance, derived from a particular plant found in this particular region, to be the instrument of his power. As a healer, Mr. Mwasapila does not need to articulate a theory of healing other than referring to the power of God. Evidently that is sufficient for a very great number of people. In performing the work of brewing the medicine in the light of a narrative telling of his relationship with God, I would argue, Mr. Mwasapila is, among other things, promising a form of security for his patients. He is bringing them into connection with the ultimate power upon whom all life depends. The implicit promise in his medicine is that access to this power will allow the patient to manage relations with the evil forces – be they viruses, cancers, evil spirits, or witchcraft, to name but a few – that are currently causing them to be sick, or may do at some time in the future. The Loliondo healer's popularity, along with testaments to his medicine's effectiveness, provides customers with confidence. The fact that he is a retired pastor probably helps, but would be less significant than evidence of his present relationship with God manifest in his success at healing the sick.

Unfortunately, for most of Mr. Mwasapila's customers this confidence that evil forces are under control will be short lived, assuming of course that none of their incurable diseases are actually cured. Before long they will begin to wonder why their suffering has not ceased. Their sense of danger, doubt, and fear regarding the invisible forces acting upon their lives will probably return, perhaps increase. When this happens, however, there will be no shortage of others promising relief to whom they can turn.

The AIDS epidemic in Africa, in tandem with the dramatic political, social, and economic changes of the past few decades, has spawned innumerable crises of authority regarding the interpretation of the actions of invisible forces in human lives. Talk of 'viruses', for example, has forced Africans to figure out how this new invisible force relates to others they have known in the past. Along with the biological ravages of the virus, itself an invisible agency, dramatic new forms of knowledge and institutions of healing – long the wellspring of religion in Africa – have spread through the continent in unprecedented ways. The AIDS epidemic has produced a widespread and pervasive sense of spiritual insecurity. Spiritual entrepreneurs of every stripe flourish amidst this insecurity. Ordinary people, too, have struggled to fashion new modes of knowing how to manage the invisible forces acting on their lives. They have been eager to embrace the promise of security. The religious enthusiasm evident across the continent is the result.

To understand phenomena such as the Loliondo Wonder or the thousands of similar events that mark the era of AIDS in Africa, we need to take seriously the narratives of power relations they embody. We need to analyse the relations spoken of in such narratives as *relations* and to take seriously the question of the politics of such relations in any particular instance, despite the fact that some of the stories we hear might seem absurd and the entities involved in the relations imaginary. The key concept here is 'spiritual insecurity'.

Spiritual insecurity emerges from relations with invisible forces (and by 'forces' I don't merely mean beings) when suffering is interpreted as harm – that is, as damage, hurt, or misfortune deliberately inflicted by malicious persons or spiritual beings.[2] Spiritual insecurity can be a cause for mere anxiety, or a matter of life and death. The struggle to find security in the face of dangers posed by invisible forces can, at times, be all consuming. By emphasising security issues, I focus on the analysis of power relations. Of course, religion, in all its multiple aspects, is about more than mere relations of power and questions of security; the quest for spiritual security, similarly, involves more than merely the religious, particularly as it involves institutions and authorities in mundane and secular domains. For most humans, however, the ultimate source of security is to be found in relations with spiritual powers of various sorts, which is why, despite reservations, I retain the term '*spiritual* insecurity' to describe this condition rather than, say 'existential' insecurity.

In this article, drawing on decades-long field experience in southern, central, and east Africa, I propose a relational realist approach to studying spiritual insecurity. By emphasising security issues, I focus on the analysis of power relations. But, crucially, I shall argue that the field of relations under analysis must include relations with and among entities beyond the merely human. Following Charles Tilly (1998, 2002), particularly in his later works, I consider that the elemental unit of human social life is the social relation – a repeated interaction between two or more persons or entities. This notion, grounding an approach to social science that Tilly called 'relational realism', stood in contradistinction to the methodological individualism, often taken-for-granted, of most social science, emphasising as it does the dispositions, motives, and calculations of individual actors. Relational realism, as performed by Tilly, also rejects the quest for governing laws to explain large social process such as war, revolution, urbanisation, class formation, and the formation of national states or responses to epidemics such as AIDS. Instead, Tilly advocated careful analysis of social relations, empirical examination of the chains of connections linking persons through time and space in larger compounds of relations. He sought to uncover the elemental logic of interactions; the causal mechanisms that recur time and again in different contexts with different results, which, he argued, could explain the dynamics of social change. Relational realism enables the social scientist to connect the actions of individuals, each constituted in relations with others, with the large processes and big structures that seem to govern their existence. Where I part company with Tilly, to some extent, is in my willingness to contemplate relations among a much wider field of entities than merely the ordinary human person.

That is to say, I propose we take seriously relations between persons and invisible entities and treat them as *relations* rather than merely as 'beliefs', a term that is seriously misused in contemporary social science (see below). While we can remain agnostic about the existence of particular parties to a relationship – say, between human and spiritual beings – and recognise thereby that we can have only a limited understanding of the relationship as it is lived, or imagined, by those engaged in it, we can nonetheless treat the relation itself as real while treating the non-human entity as virtual. Hence, this approach is a form of relational realism. Moreover, insofar as relations are treated by the persons engaged in them as relations with entities conceived of as beings or agents of some sort or another, we can analyse these relations as if they were social relations. Relations, repeated interactions between two or more entities, are far more complex and messy than the mere products of cognition and ideation known as 'beliefs'. Even if, ultimately, we are only interested in the affairs of humans, framing our understanding of their relations in this capacious way opens a much wider, more fertile, and productive field for understanding what is really going on in the world.

What is spiritual insecurity?

Merely living in a world with a lively appreciation of invisible agencies, as most humans do, does not necessarily produce spiritual insecurity. Even living with a vivid sense of exposure to evil forces in what some Christians describe as a condition of 'spiritual warfare' does not necessarily produce this insecurity. What I am calling spiritual insecurity is an existential condition marked by epistemic anxiety produced by ignorance of, uncertainty about, and/or disagreement among relevant authorities over the proper and effective modes of managing relations with agencies deemed capable of causing harm as well as those deemed responsible for the subject's safety and well-being. It is produced by crises in interpretive authority, when the people who claim to speak the truth about how the world works seem to lose persuasiveness. Insecurity mounts particularly when a superfluity of competing authorities claim the capacity to communicate and manage relations with those invisible agencies said to be responsible for causing harm – as well as those from whom protection is sought. In such circumstances people experiencing harm often face choices among conflicting authorities invoking powers rooted in radically different religious traditions, modes of ritual practice, and incompatible epistemologies. In the history of Christianity in modern Africa, for example, the central issue for Christians has been how to reconcile faith in the Biblical God and their relations with ancestors and other spirits upon whom well-being depends. Spiritual insecurity, then, is heightened by conflict among, or crises within, interpretive authorities governing relations with invisible forces, such as religious figures or healers.

Spiritual insecurity can be experienced, both individually and collectively, within a wide variety of social forms, from the solitary individual in the dead of night, to the family mourning an AIDS death together while wondering whether it was caused by witchcraft, to a whole village mobilised against Satanic bloodsuckers, or a nation reeling from a natural disasters said to have been caused by God. Although my focus in this essay is on Africa, spiritual insecurity is not a phenomenon exclusive to that continent. Yet, while the condition may be universal, the character of the relations from which it emerges – the entities experienced as being in relation, the powers they deploy, and the available modes of interpreting and managing relations – will be particular to times and places. In every context, people have to work with what we might call, with suitable homage to Charles Tilly (1977, 2008), the repertoires of spiritual action available to them, repertoires that are shaped by the particular histories of each place.

Spiritual insecurity is related to, but not reducible to, other forms of insecurity such as poverty, violence, disease, oppression, to name but a few from the UNDP's list of the components of 'human security' (1994). In the absence of manifest suffering, questions of spiritual insecurity rarely arise. Affluence and comfort give rise to their own forms of angst, to be sure, but it is in circumstances where life and death is at stake, where serious harm is feared and invisible agencies are involved that spiritual insecurity arises. The spiritual insecurity that has followed in the wake of the AIDS epidemic in Africa and that has fed the new religious enthusiasms emerges from the struggle to make sense not just of the affliction wrought by the disease, but of the conflicting schemes of interpretation propounded by medical authorities, healers, and religious leaders.

The epidemic in Africa has upended established procedures for interpreting the meaning of death. Historically, African conceptions of illness and health had no place for the notion of incurable disease, which is a condition of bodily pathology identifiable in terms of definite signs and symptoms culminating inevitably in death (Comaroff 1981, Ashforth and Nattrass 2005). Illness and health were not interpreted simply as products of biological processes, but rather as outcomes of decisions by, or struggles among, spiritual entities responsible for preserving the good in human life and those agencies – human and spiritual – seeking the destruction of the individual, his family, and community. The AIDS epidemic has not only brought the painful experience of terminal illness to multitudes in sub-Saharan Africa but also their exposure on a hitherto unseen scale to bio-medical modes of explanation and the global cultures of medical science and public health policy. In recent years, moreover, the work of interpreting the nature and meaning of illness and death has become more complicated still as anti-retroviral therapies and the news of possibilities for treating AIDS become widespread.

In sum, spiritual insecurity presents distinct epistemological problems for those experiencing it, since it emerges from uncertainty, ignorance, or disagreement over how to manage relations with invisible forces. Spiritual insecurity also poses vexing problems for those who would study it. Observers of spiritual insecurity are ordinarily unable to directly access those entities with which, or with whom, those whom they study relate, particularly those of us who dwell as secular humanists and materialists on the lonely rationalist side of the ontological divide. But though I may doubt the reality of many of the entities from which emerge the dangers, doubts, and fears I am calling spiritual insecurity, the insecurity itself is real enough, as are its consequences. How, then, might it best be studied?

Interlude: what's wrong with talking about 'beliefs'?

Before outlining a framework for the study of spiritual insecurity, let me make a case against using the concept of 'belief' in this regard. Typically, matters pertaining to what I would call spiritual insecurity are treated as questions of 'belief'. Legions of social scientists have devoted oceans of ink to describing putative 'systems of belief' within which people describe these issues. For at least half a century, however, a small number of scholars – led by Robert Bellah (1970), Rodney Needham (1972), Wilfred Cantwell Smith (1977), and Byron Good (1994) – have struggled against the tide of uncritical discourse embracing the concept 'belief'. They have mostly failed. The struggle, though futile, should continue nonetheless.[3]

There are five reasons, at least, why we should not talk about religious 'belief' and 'beliefs' in our endeavour to understand Africans' responses to AIDS. First, when social scientists refer to 'a belief' they are typically designating some spoken utterance or written sentence as a distinct propositional statement: a unit of belief. Few writers who use the word 'belief' pause to examine what the word refers to in the particular contexts about which they deploy it in their descriptions. Fewer still bother to define it. Far too many are far too naïve about the ideological underpinnings of their distinction between knowledge and belief. The term is used, even within putatively scientific discourse, as a taken-for-granted category of analysis. 'Beliefs', that is to say, are simply treated as if they are things that actually exist in the world and merely need to be discovered in any particular context.

Use of the term 'beliefs', moreover, almost always occludes systematic examination of the different kinds of propositions being advocated in various types of discourse. In most usages of 'belief', for example, writers obliterate the distinction between propositional statements that are articulated as explicit objects of belief by persons connected to human social institutions constituted through acts of faith (think of the Nicene Creed), and propositions reconstructed by observers as if they were such (think of the 'beliefs' reconstructed from answers to questions in a survey). Behind this tendency lies the history of Christian dogma – not to be mistaken, note, for those bodies of 'law' that define adherence to other religions in the Abrahamic tradition. Dogma is a comparatively tightly organised system of propositional statements to which 'believers' are supposed to actively grant credence as the foundational act of 'faith' that makes them Christian.

Propositions to be designated 'belief', whether they are reconstructions by researchers of everyday conversations to resemble the form of dogma, or actual statements by real persons designating that which is to be believed, are typically distinguished from those accorded the status of 'knowledge', usually by virtue of the institutional framework within which they are propounded. Furthermore, the distinction between knowledge and belief leaves open a huge problem concerning ignorance: how do we categorise that which our subjects don't know? Do they know not what to believe? (Which is not the same as not knowing what not to believe). Do they not know what they should? Do they wilfully refuse to believe what is true? Do they know (or think, or suspect, or fear) that a proposition is, or might be, true and still refuse to believe? As Murray Last pointed out long ago, we should never forget the 'importance of knowing about not knowing' (Last 1981).

Second, speaking of statements as "beliefs" implies that someone actually believes them. That is, that some person or persons experience an affective relation to the truth of the proposition in question – at the very least that they care, in some significant way, that the proposition be true. Very few people who write of 'beliefs', however, bother to examine, or produce evidence pertaining to, such affective relationships; instead, they merely imply that the meaning of a particular proposition labelled a 'belief' matters a lot to the person or persons who purportedly 'hold' it. As it happens, it is extremely difficult to demonstrate whether, and in what ways, a belief is believed even for a single individual, let alone a social collectivity. Again, the typical model implied in most discussions of 'belief' is that of the Christian "believer."

Preconceptions about what it means to be a believer frequently obscure analysis of *how* people believe when they believe themselves to be believing something. When making claims about the 'holding' of 'beliefs', most observers merely reconstruct utterances as if they were elements of a dogma, or, worse, the preconceptions that purportedly underpin utterances reconstructed to resemble dogma. Few analysts ever bother to examine *how* putative believers believe, or struggle against believing, such reconstructed sets of propositions. In research on AIDS in Africa, for example, how extensive is the literature on *akrasia* of belief, the failure of the will to resist believing something a persons knows she should not believe (such as the proposition that witchcraft can cause AIDS; Ashforth 2005)? It is virtually non-existent. Rather than presuming some *thing* to exist within a person's mind, a belief he can have and hold, it would be better, it seems to me, to listen to what people say.

Third, talk of 'beliefs' generally presumes that particular propositional statements exist as elements of a putative 'system of beliefs' in which a set of 'beliefs' are logically interrelated. Yet again, the implicit model here is the Western Christian phenomenon of dogma. Dogma, as it happens, was – and still is – written down. Systems of belief outside of written texts designed for such relations, and their corpus of exegetical writings, may, or may not, exist. That is an empirical question. It would be hard, I fear, for someone schooled in the 'Western' tradition of distinguishing tradition from modernity or the popular from the established to distinguish whether what his informant is telling him is really part of a 'system' of beliefs. Writers who refer to such systems and their related 'structures of belief', rarely bother to demonstrate the systematicity of their putative 'system', let alone how the existence of such a system can be determined as a product of the utterances of mere humans, blathering away as we are wont. Beyond the bounds of institutions governed by authorities entrusted with enshrining specific holy texts and ritual practices with an expectation of credence, it is extremely difficult to demonstrate the existence among ordinary people leading ordinary lives that a 'system of belief' exists, or describe what it is, and explain in what sense it is systematic.

Fourth, those who write and talk of 'systems of belief' tend to presume that this entity maps in some way, usually unspecified, onto particular individual minds, and, what turns out to be the same thing, some social collectivity treated as if it were an individual mind. Ordinarily, 'a system of belief' is treated as a synonym for '*a culture*' (a concept usually defined in terms of a shared system of values, attitudes, and beliefs within some socially bounded collectivity). Social psychologists, who have dominated research in the social science of AIDS in Africa, tend to do this reflexively on account of their methodological individualism. Despite an increasing awareness of the complexity of questions of identity, however, many social researchers who should know better do the same. Anthropology, which was an enterprise built upon the promise of deciphering a collectivity's 'culture' by means of a few conversations with representative members thereof, has long ago recognised the futility of the endeavour to find and describe a bounded culture (Geertz 2000). Habits, however, are hard to break. Few researchers who now bear the burden of 'culture' in their efforts to explain 'behaviour' bother to engage with the empirical question of whether the 'belief system' at issue really belongs to the particular collectivity under study in any meaningful sense. It is theoretically possible to do this, but difficult and expensive. Specialists in market research are making some headway in demonstrating when and how this occurs, with a view to selling products. I doubt, which is to say I do not believe, that this methodology will soon make much headway in revealing things that matter in relation to AIDS and religion in Africa.

Fifth, talk of 'beliefs' carries another embedded presumption that is rarely subjected to critical scrutiny or supported with empirical evidence: that the propositional statement so labelled serves as a motive to, or governs in some sense, action. Again, we are dealing with a legacy of Western Christendom in this usage of the term belief. In the universe of propositions that may be uttered, those that are presumed to matter when we talk about believing, resonate in, refer to, or emerge from something that has come to be known as the Conscience. Yet, as anyone who has tried to accurately account for the relation between what a person says and what he does will know, whether from experience in the courtroom or the bedroom, this is difficult work. Rather than presuming a connection between particular propositional statements and actions, it seems to me, the social researcher should examine the various forms of connection between thought, talk, and action in particular contexts.

Rather than proceed with an uncritical usage of 'belief', then, let me stipulate a few simple rules for analysis of narrative and discourse. We should start by always seeking to specify who says what, to whom, where, when, how, and why? We should examine the ways in which narratives are constructed in order to identify common patterns and reveal the predicates underpinning their meaningfulness. Further, we should examine the statements made in narratives explaining and justifying action. We should try to identify the implicit rules underpinning the making of valid statements in conversations and debates including claims about 'belief'. (These usually become clearer in the breech). We should examine the assumptions and predicates underpinning statements that serve as valid. And we should inquire into the conditions of plausibility governing these assumptions. Plausibility, I take to be the condition of being believable. It is far easier to demonstrate that a proposition is believable, by analysis of the context of life within which it might be stated without provoking efforts at refutation, as well as the presuppositions that logically underpin its possibility of being stated, than that it is actually 'believed' in some person's putative mental state. It is also easier to demonstrate how certain propositions gain or lose plausibility than to explain why persons might have changed, or not changed, the things in which they believe.

A relational realist framework for the analysis of spiritual insecurity in Africa in the time of AIDS

Security is a relational concept. Whatever it is that we talk about when we talk about security and its absence, we are referring to a feature of relations, more specifically power relations with human persons and other entities intent on causing harm. Thus, proper analysis of conditions of security and insecurity requires broad examination of the power relations within which people live – or think they live. Where people see themselves as living in relations with invisible beings and powers, which is almost everywhere, failure to take account of these relations as social relations, rather than mere beliefs, will prevent a proper understanding of the questions of security relevant to that particular context.

For the analysis of spiritual insecurity, in Africa and elsewhere, four broad sets of relations require examination.

First, analysis must resolve questions of relations among persons as ordinarily understood in the specific context, particularly in terms of their putative access to occult powers. These powers are usually classified under the rubrics 'witchcraft' and 'sorcery' and are typically said to derive from inherent capacities, secret knowledge, or relations with invisible beings – or some combination of each. Presumptions regarding the motives of otherwise normal persons for using occult power are typically spoken of as hatred, jealousy, and the desire for illicit wealth and power. Most Africans also know a category of persons – conveniently translated as the English word 'witch', though known by a variety of local terms across the continent – who are deemed so devoted to the pursuit of evil through the use of supernatural powers they no longer remain truly human.

The predicament of living in a world with witches, such as I have tried to describe in my work on Soweto, can sometimes surprise those of us who have not grown up in such places and can produce much misunderstanding. Because of witchcraft, a presumption of malice underpins community life. You must presume witches will harm you because they can. If they choose to kill you with AIDS, they might contrive by mystical means for you to contract HIV from a sex partner. If you already have AIDS and a witch wishes to kill you his task is made simpler and the crime of witchcraft will be harder to detect (which is another reason people say you should be circumspect in talking openly about the disease). They might also kill you with a man-made disease, witchcraft fabricated to look like AIDS though without traces of HIV infection. You never know. Anyone who has experienced what witches can do, will know that no one can say for sure that such things are impossible.

A central fact of life in the parts of Africa I know is that when a misfortune such as the illness unto death that is AIDS strikes, people are forced by all the weight of custom and existential dread to face the question: who is to blame? It is impossible to tell a satisfying story of death without imputing responsibility to someone. Talk of AIDS, in which blame is usually attributed either to the victim or a sexual partner, takes place within contexts shaped by older practices of attributing responsibility, notably witchcraft. AIDS discourse does not supplant witchcraft discourse in narratives of illness and death but becomes another resource in the micro-politics of suspicion and accusation. For people who need to know the 'real' reasons for an illness, however, the competing frames of interpretation provided by different types of healers can prove utterly destabilising. The advent of anti-retroviral therapy with dramatic mortality declines in some parts of the continent has changed this dynamic to some extent, though it remains to be seen what the long-term impact will be.

The AIDS epidemic in Africa has brought massive new misfortunes to families and communities where the fear of human access to supernatural occult powers is pervasive. An 'epistemological double bind', then, pervades relationships with neighbours, colleagues, and kin (Ashforth 2005). Since you can discount neither the motive (his jealousy and hatred can be deeply hidden) nor the capacity (anything is possible) of the witch, you should be distrustful of all, always. As my friend Madumo was fond of saying of life in a world with witches, it is 'exposed' (Ashforth 2000). The danger of occult assault is ever-present, though not always expected – witchcraft is almost always experienced as a surprise. Most of the time occult dangers are more or less manageable. The most successful religious movements and entrepreneurs in contemporary Africa are those promising protection from occult assault. Huge amounts of time, energy, and money, however, are invested in this business and have been for generations. In recent decades these have to a large extent been channelled into enthusiastic religious movements such as Pentecostalism.

Second, the analysis needs to properly frame questions pertaining to relations between persons and the powers inherent in substances (particularly substances such as medicines and poisons presumed to possess agency, but also inert polluting substances); images (particularly images of human persons and spiritual beings); objects (both embodying or representing invisible powers); and texts (particularly books, a sort of talismanic hybrid of image and object, containing the word of God). This is a massive field of inquiry, hugely dynamic, and I shall not begin to survey it here.[4] Understandings of these relations in the places where I work are constantly changing, sometimes rapidly. For example, in many parts of Africa a notion of 'African Science' has become a primary frame of plausibility governing supposition about the powers of witches and sorcerers to manipulate the powers inherent in substance in order to cause harm (Ashforth 2005). Similar presumptions are at work in the commonplace talk of traditional healing as 'science', and the related investment, particularly in post-apartheid South Africa, in demonstrating the scientific basis of supposedly 'traditional' remedies. Everyday experience of technologies such as computers, cell-phones, and the remote control have made suppositions regarding relations with powerful substances more plausible to young people, though in a new register. Science, that is to say, shows few signs of driving out superstition.

African talk about the powers in substances both harmful and health-giving should not be mistaken for a form of elementary pharmacology. Remember the story of the healer in Loliondo dispensing medicine made from the 'mugagira' tree. As he made clear in numerous interviews, the active force in the medicine was the power of God. To be effective, moreover, the decoction had to be dispensed by the healer's hand directly. The efficacy of this substance, then, is a product of relations among God, the healer, some active element in the brew, and the set of forces producing whatever it is that ails a patient. The actual bioactive properties of the substance are almost beside the point. Indeed, many healing churches omit the herbs and work solely with water and prayer.

When interpreting the ways people make sense of and manage relations with the forces they see operating in the world around them, we must be wary of presuming systematicity and stability. My experience in this field convinces me that a profusion of confusion is the norm, rather than neat and tidy 'systems of belief'. Recent decades in Africa, as elsewhere, have seen a proliferation of interpretive authorities, people claiming to know the truth about invisible forces and the ability to manage relations with them, particularly healers and religious entrepreneurs offering access to miraculous substances or holy words and images capable of delivering miraculous healing. Perhaps the most significant substance to enter the scene in recent years has been the 'ARV', a substance whose agency and modes of action is not easy to understand in any language.[5] A popular term for ARVs has emerged recently in Malawi where they are referred to as 'maUnits' by analogy to the ubiquitous prepaid cell phone units for sale on every street corner. Similar terminology, I suspect, can be found elsewhere. They are used, I am told, to 'top up life'.

Third, we need a better way of analysing the politics of power relations among invisible beings and between persons and invisible beings than is currently available under the rubric 'belief'. These relations can conduce to a sense of insecurity as well as being the foundation, for most people, of their sense of security in the face of invisible forces intent on harm. Ritual, for example, on which there is a massive literature in Africa as elsewhere, almost always involves communing between ordinary persons and invisible beings. Dance, trance, and the wide expanse of otherworldly out-of-body experiences make these relations seem real. Watch the trembling, shaking, shrieking, and falling that goes on during a Deliverance Service in a Born Again church, when demons are driven out and the sick cured, and you will see the bodiliness of these relations with invisible beings. Insecurity arises in this domain when people are torn between competing interpretations of the nature and intentions of invisible beings with whom they experience relations, or find themselves ignorant of how to supplicate unto spiritual powers and protect themselves from evil agencies. It can also arise when the moral nature of invisible beings with whom people experience relationships – in all the emotional intensity and bodily presence that such being are known to dispose – is cast into doubt.

The two central questions about relations with invisible beings that AIDS confronts Africans with are: to what extent is God and other entities responsible for the suffering and death (and why has He, or they, done this?); and: how do we access the power of spiritual beings to heal the sick and protect against injury? It is a commonplace of everyday discourse throughout the continent, for example, that God is punishing Africa with AIDS (Behrend 2007). Many preachers and theologians try to teach otherwise, though with limited success (Bongmba 2007). At the same time, legions of preachers are at work proclaiming the news that God, through the Holy Spirit can perform miracles of healing (and that they, by virtue of their spiritual powers can help their followers access that power). Across the continent there is an enormous ferment of religious activity, most notably in the form of Pentecostalism (Kalu 2008), that I would argue is in large part a response to spiritual insecurity, much of which is a response to AIDS.

Religious faith, I should emphasise, is not in itself the source of the insecurity I am describing as 'spiritual'. Spiritual insecurity, however, cannot arise in the absence of faith; it flourishes in the space between faith and doubt, for without faith there would be no relationship about which one might worry. The new religious movements of Africa are alike in their insistence of certainty in their relations with invisible beings, though they wreak havoc with older ways of managing relations with spiritual beings, and not only in the realm of the 'traditional' (Engelke 2010). Nowhere is this more evident than in Pentecostal preachers' demonisation, literally, of ancestors as evil spirits and denunciation of their veneration as 'idol worship' (Muller and De Villiers 1987). This at a time when older missionary Christian denominations are striving to incorporate African 'traditions' into their rituals and theology (Bate 1995). 'Born Agains', it should be noted, have a similar repugnance for Catholicism's saints. But the increasing obsession with Satan and his demons that is common across Africa, along with the enthusiasm for 'deliverance' that countless preachers are harvesting, brings a danger similar to that long experienced by traditional healers who faced suspicions of witchcraft: one man's Spirit-filled miracle working pastor is another's devil worshipping Satanist.[6]

Fourth, and finally, in order to understand the dimensions of spiritual insecurity in any given place, we need to understand relations among the internal agencies said by people there to be internal to, and constitutive of, their sense of being alive, their 'personhood' as it is sometimes called. Among the entities ordinarily said to be in action within the self, such as body, mind, spirit, soul, will, etc. – the list could go on – a new one has come on the scene in Africa recently: the immune system. For those of us schooled in the quaint notions of modern individualism, it can be hard to appreciate how others might understand the constituent elements of their selves as being capable of action independent of their 'will', or, more problematic still, how these agencies might interact with other agencies beyond the purview of a person's perception and consciousness, let alone control. Think about dreams. Those of us accustomed to living in the dull sublunary realms of Western modernity tend to conceive of dreams as phenomena internal to the mind of an individual, products of the functioning of a brain. We tend not to think of the dream world as a domain of action wherein agents of one sort and another, such as the manifold internal essences of human personhood (of the dead as well as the living), along with spirits, demons, deities, and what have you, interact with each other and actually do things – real things that have concrete repercussions in the waking world.[7]

I would describe relations among constitutive elements of personhood in political terms involving power relations. This 'politics of personhood' can produce what might be termed 'vulnerabilities of the soul'. Vulnerability, I should mention, is not the same as insecurity. A healer who opens himself to the agency of spirits in his work of healing while certainly vulnerable, need not necessarily be experiencing spiritual insecurity. A man, who fears he has been doctored with love medicine such as *korobela*, which hijack his sexual desire and make him vulnerable to feelings of love, probably is. Vulnerability generates insecurity in the light of the presumption of malice regarding the motives of others. Love medicine, for example, when deployed by a wife against her husband can make him her slave, blind to her sexual infidelities, and thus at risk of HIV infection – or so I've heard men in Malawi argue. (Women, on the other hand, can argue that such stuff, known locally as *konda ine*, can protect a faithful wife from being infected by binding the husband to his home and marital bed, regardless of his will or faithless desires.)[8]

The point of this brief survey of some of the possibilities imagined in contemporary Africa as power relations from which a sense of insecurity can emerge in the context of AIDS is to underline the fundamental fact that for the vast majority of people, a sense of security derives primarily from relations with those invisible beings that are usually referred to as 'spiritual'. Hence, the importance of understanding spiritual insecurity.

Conclusion: AIDS and religious enthusiasm

In the decades since AIDS began ravaging the continent, Africa has witnessed an efflorescence of religious enthusiasm. New Christian and Islamic movements have flourished as Africans embrace global religious organisations and export their own brand of enthusiasm to global markets. Religious entrepreneurs bearing novel doctrines and extravagant promises are everywhere to be found. Healers proliferate, marketing their 'medicines' with a mixture of 'science' and 'spirit'. Preachers promise prosperity. On banners stretched across roads, paintings on the sides of shops and vehicles, simple signs perched atop poles or painted on rocks – anywhere, it seems, that words can be written – the landscape of the continent is littered with advertisements for salvation. Everywhere people seem obsessed with demons, witches, and occult forces. Enormous amounts of time, energy, and money are being invested in efforts to secure protection from supernatural dangers.

This efflorescence of religious enthusiasm has been roughly coterminous with the AIDS epidemic. The question this paper addresses is: how are we to understand the connection?[9]

For reasons that remain obscure, though if Darwin is any guide probably have to do with survival of the species, humans seem to have evolved a sense – we might call it a conviction – that their security depends upon agencies and entities that are sometimes described, amongst a plethora of possible terms, as supernatural, extra-human, spiritual, or invisible. Most people, in most places, to paraphrase a former senior adviser to President George W. Bush, seem not to live in 'reality-based communities' (Suskind 2004). Realists ignore this fact at their peril. And while a suspicion has recently emerged among a small elite of the species over the past couple of centuries that such convictions are merely products of the human mind, a form of belief, and thus irreducibly subjective, most people throughout what we know of the history of humanity, have lived in ways that are premised upon the objectivity of these entities and the forces they embody.

Conventionally, these matters are discussed under rubric 'religion'. Such a framing, however, narrows the issue by tying it too closely to the concept of belief, and its cousin faith (Bellah 1970, Smith 1977). A better solution, this paper has argued, is to open the analysis of power relations, upon which human security ultimately depends, to include relations with other agencies and entities beyond the merely human. This is not as outlandish as it might sound.

Notes

1. Space precludes a comprehensive review of the literatures relating to healing and religion here. For a good recent survey of literature pertaining to religion, see Harri Englund's introduction to Englund (2011). And for a good recent survey of the literature on healing in Africa, see Manglos and Trinitapoli (2011).
2. It is beyond the scope of this paper to why suffering is experienced as harm. Suffice it to say that the ethnographic record of Africa, exemplified by the enormous literature on witchcraft, is replete with examples showing *that* this is the case. For a survey of this literature, see Moore and Sanders (2001).
3. Space precludes detailed critique of the large number of publications that are drawn on here. Instead I commend the reader to a single paper, which exemplifies the errors catalogued below. See Kalichman and Simbayi (2004).
4. For a more detailed elaboration, see (Ashforth 2005; Pt 2).
5. For a discussion of an effort to translate the action of ARVs into 'culturally relevant' terms, see Ashforth and Nattrass (2005).
6. Nowhere is this more evident than in attitudes to the enormously successful Brazilian church the Universal Church of the Kingdom of God. See Van Wyk (2011).
7. For a classic ethnographical description of what can be accomplished in dreams, see Evans-Pritchard (1937).
8. For a study of these 'herbs' in Zimbabwe, see Goebel (2002).
9. This period has also seen major political and economic transformations in Africa such as structural adjustment and democratisation, which have also impacted on religious life, but I shall not touch on these here. For a good account of the more general field, see Ellis and Ter Haar (2004).

References

Ashforth, A., 2000. *Madumo, a man bewitched*. Chicago, IL: University of Chicago Press.

Ashforth, A., 2005. *Witchcraft, violence, and democracy in South Africa*. Chicago, IL: University of Chicago Press.

Ashforth, A. and Nattrass, N., 2005. Ambiguities of 'culture' and antiretroviral rollout in South Africa. *Social Dynamics*, 31 (2), 285–303.

Bate, S.C., 1995. *Inculturation and healing: coping-healing in South African Christianity*. Pietermaritzburg: Cluster Publications.

Behrend, H., 2007. The rise of occult powers, AIDS and the Roman Catholic Church in Western Uganda. *Journal of Religion in Africa*, 37, 41–58.

Behrend, H. and Luig, U., 1999. *Spirit possession, modernity, and power in Africa*. Oxford/Kampala/Cape Town/Madison: James Currey/Fountain Publishers/David Philip/University of Wisconsin Press.

Bellah, R.N., 1970. *Beyond belief: essays on religion in a post-traditional world*. New York: Harper and Row.

Bongmba, E.K., 2007. Facing a pandemic: the African church and the crisis of HIV/AIDS. Waco, TX: Baylor University Press.

Comaroff, J., 1981. Healing and the cultural order: the case of the Barolong boo Ratshidi of Southern Africa. *American Ethnologist*, 7 (4), 637–657.

Doran, M.C.M., 2007. Reconstructing Mchape '95: AIDS, Billy Chisupe, and the politics of persuasion. *Journal of Eastern African Studies*, 1 (3), 397–416.

Ellis, S. and Ter Haar, G., 2004. *Worlds of power: religious thought and political practice in Africa*. New York: Oxford University Press.

Engelke, M., 2010. Past Pentecostalism: notes on rupture, realignment, and everyday life in Pentecostal and African Independent Churches. *Africa (London 1928)*, 80 (2), 177–199.

Englund, H., ed., 2011. *Christianity and public culture in Africa*. Athens: Ohio University Press.

Evans-Pritchard, E.E., 1937. *Witchcraft oracles and magic among the Azande*. Oxford: Clarendon Press.

Geertz, C., 2000. The world in pieces: culture and politics at the end of the century. *In*: C. Geertz, ed. *Available light: anthropological reflections on philosophical topics*. Princeton, NJ: Princeton University Press, 218–263.

Goebel, A., 2002. 'Men these days, they are a problem': husband-taming herbs and gender wars in rural Zimbabwe. *Canadian Journal of African Studies/Revue Canadienne des Études Africaines*, 36 (3), 460–489.

Good, B., 1994. *Medicine, rationality, and experience*. Cambridge: Cambridge University Press.

Guardian-on-Sunday-Team, 2011. Journey to Loliondo's Magic Man. *Guardian on Sunday (Tanzania)*. Dar es Salaam. Available from: http://www.ippmedia.com/frontend/index. php?l=26953 [Accessed 28 July 2011].

Hume, D., 1963 [1742–1754]. Of superstition and enthusiasm. *In*: D. Hume, ed. *Essays, moral, political, and literary*. Oxford: Oxford University Press.

Kalichman, S.C. and Simbayi, L., 2004. Traditional beliefs about the cause of AIDS and AIDS-related stigma in South Africa. *AIDS Care*, 16 (5), 572–580.

Kalu, O., 2008. African Pentecostalism: an introduction. Oxford: Oxford University Press.

Kalu, O.U., 2009. A discursive interpretation of African Pentecostalism. *Fides et historia*, 41 (1), 71.

Knox, R.A., 1950. *Enthusiasm: a chapter in the history of religion with special reference to the XVII and XVIII centuries*. Oxford: Oxford University Press.

Last, M., 1981. The importance of knowing about not knowing. *Social Science and Medicine*, 15 (3B), 387–392.

Manglos, N.D. and Trinitapoli, J., 2011. The third therapeutic system: faith healing strategies in the context of a generalized AIDS epidemic. *Journal of Health and Social Behavior*, 52 (1), 107–122.

Moore, H. and Sanders, T., eds. 2001. Magical interpretations and material realities: an introduction. *In*: *Magical interpretations, material realities: modernity, witchcraft and the occult in postcolonial Africa*. London: Routledge, 1–27.

Muller, F.P. and De Villiers, P., 1987. *Pentecostal perspectives on the activity of demonic powers. Like a roaring lion … Essays on the Bible, the church and demonic powers*. Pretoria South Africa: C.B. Powell Bible Centre, 173–191.

Needham, R., 1972. *Belief, language, and experience*. Chicago, IL: University of Chicago Press.

Nation Television (NTV) Kenya, 2011. *The Loliondo Wonder*. March 22, 23. Available from: http://www.youtube.com/watch?v=iKOwDQcPwbs

Pew Forum, 2010. *Tolerance and tension: Islam and Christianity in Sub-Saharan Africa*. West Conshohocken, PA: Pew Forum for Religion and Public Life.

Probst, P., 1999. 'Mchape '95', or, the sudden fame of Billy Goodson Chisupe: healing, social memory and the enigma of the public sphere in Post-Banda Malawi. *Africa (London 1928)*, 69 (1), 108–137.

Schoffeleers, M., 1999. The AIDS pandemic, the prophet Billy Chisupe, and the democratization process in Malawi. *Journal of Religion in Africa*, 29 (4), 406–441.

Smith, W.C., 1977. *Belief and history*. Charlottesburg: University of Virginia Press.

Suskind, R., 2004. Faith, certainty, and the presidency of George W. Bush. *New York Times Magazine*. October 17.

Tilly, C., 1977. Getting it together in Burgundy, 1675–1975. *Theory and Society*, 4, 479–504.

Tilly, C., 1998. *Micro, macro, or Megrim? In*: J. Schlumbohm, ed. *Mikrogeschichte – Makrogeschichte: komplementär oder inkommensurabel?* Göttingen: Wallstein Verlag, 7.

Tilly, C., 2002. *Stories, identities, and political change*. Lanham, MD: Rowman and Littlefield.

Tilly, C., 2008. *Contentious performances*. Cambridge: Cambridge University Press.

Tucker, S.I., 1972. *Enthusiasm; a study in semantic change*. Cambridge: Cambridge University Press.

UNDP, 1994. *Human development report 1994*. New York/Oxford: Oxford University Press for the United Nations Development Programme.

Van Wyk, I., 2011. Believing practically and trusting socially: the contrary case of the Universal Church of the Kingdom of God in Durban, South Africa. *In*: H. Englund, ed. *Christianity and public culture in Africa*. Athens: University of Ohio Press, 189–203.

Fighting down the scourge, building up the church: Organisational constraints in religious involvement with HIV/AIDS in Mozambique

Victor Agadjanian and Cecilia Menjívar

School of Social and Family Dynamics, Arizona State University, Tempe, Arizona, USA

Religious organisations (ROs) are often said to play an important role in mitigating the impact of HIV/AIDS. Yet, limitations of that role have also been acknowledged. While most of the literature has focused on ideological and individual-level implications of religion for HIV/AIDS, in this study we shift the focus to the organisational factors that shape and constrain ROs' involvement in both HIV prevention and HIV/AIDS care and support. Using primarily qualitative data collected in a predominantly Christian area in southern Mozambique, we show that the organisational vitality of a RO as determined by its membership size and its relationships with other churches and with governmental and non-governmental agencies is a pervasive priority of RO leaders. Therefore, all church activities, including those related to HIV/AIDS, are instrumentalised by the religious leadership to achieve the church's organisational aims – maintaining and growing its membership, safeguarding the often precarious coexistence with other churches, and enhancing its standing vis-à-vis the government and powerful non-governmental organisations. As a result, the effectiveness of ROs' involvement in HIV/AIDS prevention and assistance is often compromised.

Background and conceptual approach

Religious organisations (ROs) are often said to play an important role in mitigating the impact of the HIV/AIDS epidemic in resource-limited settings (Tiendrebeogo and Bukyx 2004, Olivier *et al.* 2006, Becker and Geissler 2009, Chitando 2010). Public accounts of that role typically stress ROs' unique ideological and organisational advantages for community mobilisation and outreach as well as a long-established tradition of faith-based provision of health care and psychological support to the disadvantaged masses, especially in rural areas. However, many of these public accounts are anecdotal and come from ROs and other faith-based organisations and therefore seldom rely on systematic and impartial analyses of ROs' activities (Byamugisha *et al.* 2002, Bate 2003). Moreover, these accounts are often produced by the religious officialdom that is typically based in national capitals and other large cities and whose target audience is governmental and non-governmental funding agencies. Voices of local religious leaders, not to mention ROs' rank-and-file members, are rarely heard.

The scholarly literature on the role of ROs in mitigating the impact of HIV/AIDS is generally less celebratory, and studies have identified several problematic areas that are inherent to most ROs or vary in importance across different types of ROs (Trinitapoli and Regnerus 2006, Agadjanian and Sen 2007, Haddad *et al.* 2008, Francis and Liverpool 2009, Trinitapoli 2009, Casale *et al.* 2010). Thus it has been argued that ROs may contribute to HIV/AIDS-related stigma and discrimination (Mbilinyi and Kaihula 2000, Regnerus and Salinas 2007, Zou *et al.* 2009, Keikelame *et al.* 2010). Perhaps one of the most frequently discussed issues is many ROs' critical or ambivalent stance and practice in regards to condom use (Garner 2000a, Pfeiffer 2004, Casale *et al.* 2010).

Whereas the position of some religious leaders on HIV prevention has aroused occasional controversy, ROs' role in the provision of psychological support, home care and even material aid to AIDS-affected individuals and families is usually described in strongly positive terms (Trinitapoli 2006, Maman *et al.* 2009). The range and magnitude of ROs' activities aimed at helping the sick, the dying and the survivors, especially in settings where few viable alternatives are available, deserve considerable praise. However, challenges that ROs may face in carrying out these activities have also been noted (Agadjanian and Sen 2007, Krakauer and Newbery 2007, Watt *et al.* 2009).

The objective of this study is to explore ROs' HIV/AIDS related-activities in a resource-limited setting through an organisational lens. While acknowledging and documenting different forms of ROs' involvement in HIV/AIDS prevention and care, we start by highlighting factors, both internal and external to ROs, that shape and constrain the organisational parameters of this involvement. These factors are demographics of RO membership, ROs' access to financial and material resources, ROs' uneasy coexistence and interactions in an increasingly crowded and saturated religious marketplace, and ROs' complex relationship with secular authorities and institutions. We then examine how organisational pressures rooted in these factors affect ROs' involvement in HIV prevention and in HIV/AIDS-related care and support. We look at prevention and care/support separately because the nature, meaning, and ideological and organisational ramifications of these two types of activities are sufficiently distinct in sub-Saharan settings. However, both types of activities are necessarily interconnected, not only because they revolve around the same broad theme – HIV infection and disease – but also because both, as we intend to show, are part of ROs' efforts to enhance their organisational vitality. We therefore argue that in order to evaluate what ROs do or do not do to help fight the HIV/AIDS epidemic, one must first understand how HIV/AIDS-related activities help ROs in meeting their organisational needs.

Data and method

This case study focuses on Mozambique, a nation of some 23 million inhabitants in south-east Africa that gained independence from Portugal in 1975, lived through a devastating civil war in 1977–1992, and despite political stability and strong macroeconomic growth since the war ended, remains one of the poorest in the world. The data used in this study were collected in Chibuto district, a largely rural area in Gaza province in southern Mozambique. The traditional lineage system of the Changana, the ethnic group that constitutes the overwhelming majority of the district's population, is patrilineal and their marriage is virilocal. The mainstay of the area's economy is subsistence agriculture. The low and unpredictable yields, the lack of local non-agricultural employment and the proximity to South Africa have resulted in high levels of primarily male labour out-migration. This large-scale migration may have contributed to the area's high HIV prevalence. While no district-level HIV prevalence estimates are available, HIV prevalence in Gaza province as a whole was estimated at 25% of the adult population in 2009, the highest seroprevalence level of all Mozambican provinces (Ministry of Health 2010, p. 163).

Our analysis draws primarily from focus group discussions held in Chibuto district in 2009. Seven focus groups were carried out: two in the town of Chibuto, the district's capital, and one in each of the district's five administrative posts (subdivisions). Focus groups participants were selected from different local ROs to represent a wide denominational spectrum. All focus group participants were RO rank-and-file members – members with formal leadership duties were not eligible for participation. The number of participants ranged between 6 and 16 per group. The five focus group discussions conducted outside the district capital were gender-mixed; in the district capital, one group included only men and the other only women. In total, 74 individuals, 44 women and 30 men, participated in the focus group discussions. The discussions revolved primarily around ROs' activities in areas of HIV education and prevention and provision of care and support to individuals and families affected by HIV/AIDS. The focus group data are used to identify and explore organisational imperatives and constraints in district religious organisations' involvement in these activities.

To provide a background for the analysis, we also use data from a household-based survey conducted in Chibuto in 2008 and an institutional survey of religious congregations carried out in the district in 2008–2009. The sample of the household-based survey consisted of 2019 women aged 18–50 drawn from the population of both the district capital and the five administrative posts. The survey included questions on women's sociodemographic characteristics, religious background and involvement, and on HIV/AIDS-related matters, among other questions. The institutional survey covered all ROs operating in the district ($N = 811$) and consisted of interviews with RO leaders that were focused on congregation characteristics and activities. Both surveys included similar questions on whether RO leaders had addressed HIV/AIDS-related topics during religious services in the several preceding months: in the women's survey questionnaire, a list of specific topics was provided; in the institutional survey, respondents were asked to name all the specific HIV/AIDS-related topics that they could remember. Finally, the analysis includes insights and observations from the authors' numerous interviews and conversations with RO leaders and members alike to illustrate the ideological and organisational narratives employed in navigating ROs' involvement in HIV prevention and AIDS-related care and support.

Organisational dynamics in the religious marketplace

The Chibuto district, like the rest of Mozambique and much of sub-Saharan Africa, is characterised by high levels of religious membership. Thus 88% of the 2008 survey respondents reported being affiliated with a RO. The district's religious population is overwhelmingly Christian, with denominations ranging from the Roman Catholic

Church (the dominant church before Mozambique's independence), to mainline, or mission-based, Protestant and Evangelical denominations (e.g., Presbyterian, Methodist, Anglican, Baptist), to international Pentecostal churches, to regionally initiated Apostolic churches, to locally grown owner-operated Pentecostal (Zionist) churches. The institutional survey included only two mosques and less than 1% of the women's survey respondents with a religious affiliation were Muslim. Besides, almost all Chibuto Muslims live in the district's administrative capital. Hence this analysis is focused entirely on Christian churches.

Based on our survey data, we estimate that there is approximately one congregation for every 150–200 adult district residents, although congregations vary by membership size and attendance. The small pool of unaffiliated people and the saturation of the religious marketplace reduce the prospects for proselytising. Although the relatively rapid population growth provides a supply of new potential members, this supply cannot satisfy the demands of ever multiplying churches and their leaders' desire to expand their ranks. Religious organisation leaders are therefore extremely vigilant about protecting their turf, and any venturing outside its limits for whatever stated reason can be interpreted as an attempt to 'steal believers' from other churches. The threat of losing members to other churches, while often downplayed by religious leaders, is nonetheless omnipresent. The threat comes, at least potentially, from other congregations operating in the same area as well as from outside-the-district ROs, which are mainly headquartered in Maputo, Mozambique's capital city a couple hundred kilometres to the south, and are relatively well-heeled financially and institutionally. These outsiders, typically led by entrepreneurial pastors, encroach, often quite aggressively, on the already established and apportioned religious territory thus generating resentment and even overt hostility on the part of local religious leaders.

Raising funds for congregation needs and activities is a constant concern of RO leaders. Importantly, while leaders of large mainline congregations often receive a salary and living allowance (however modest) from their churches, most leaders of smaller, Pentecostal and Apostolic congregations have to support themselves. Leaders of such congregations are therefore under constant pressure to generate funds for the congregation operational budget and capital investments (e.g., church building construction) and often for their personal needs. Although most of these leaders hold formal or informal income-generating jobs and are typically better off than most district residents, their individual incomes are not sufficient to cover the church needs. Most RO funds come from congregation members, whose value to the congregation is therefore largely determined by their ability and willingness to make regular and substantial financial contributions. In addition, a substantial portion of Apostolic and Pentecostal ROs' revenues come from the provision of healing services both to congregation members and to non-members. Miracle healing is a trademark specialty of Zionist congregations: 76% of Zionist leaders interviewed in the institutional survey answered affirmatively the question 'Do they usually cure illnesses in your church?' Although no fixed fees are usually charged for treatment (with the exception of the costs of the traditional medicines when such are used), the patients and their families are expected to 'thank' the pastor either in money or in kind (or both). Whereas Pentecostal pastors are typically eager to maximise this revenue stream, unsuccessful treatment may undermine their credibility inside and outside the congregation, while excessive marketing of healing services outside the congregation carries a potential for inter-church frictions.

Partly to reduce the possibility of potential clashes and partly to pool individual ROs' material and political resources, several inter-church coordinating bodies have been established. The Christian Council (the local branch of a national outfit) that brings together most mainline Protestant denominations was founded before Mozambique's independence and is perhaps the oldest of them. In comparison, the Organisation of Zionist Pentecostal Churches of Mozambique, known by its Portuguese acronym 'OISPM' was created just a few years ago. Its regional branch, with membership in Chibuto and other neighbouring districts, organise a sort of rotating credit scheme among its members modelled after the widespread practice of individual resource-pooling locally known as *xitique*. The main purpose of this organisational xitique is to assist churches in building or improving their houses of worship; in fact, instead of money, bags of cement are usually distributed. However, as our interviews and observations showed, the OISPM is fraught with conflict and distrust as each cycle of money collection and distribution generates suspicions of unfairness, favouritism and even fraud on the part of the organisation's leaders. The transfer of some of the funds raised through members' annual quotas to the organisation's headquarters in Maputo has also raised discontent. As a result, an increasing number of RO leaders that are nominally part of OISPM refuse to contribute to the organisation's coffers.

Another important factor that local RO leaders take into account is their relationship with the government. There are several types of ties that ROs seek to establish and cultivate. The District has a Commission for Religious Affairs (a branch of the national agency that is part of the Department of Justice). Although the authority of the Commission is limited and largely ceremonial, it is part of the government apparatus and its leadership has close ties with the office of the District's Administrator. For example, it is the Commission's chairman who usually reads the inaugural prayer with which almost all district-level public events, however secular in nature, invariably start. However, the Commission represents but one link between ROs and the government. Other connections with state institutions at both the district and, especially, the sub-district (administrative post, locality and village) levels are also important and take a variety of forms. Many of them are personal and unofficial: for example, a local administrator, health official or school principal may double as a church pastor. Religious organization leaders using their connections, authority, education and organisational and rhetorical skills may also establish local non-governmental organisations (NGOs) or become local managers of regional and national NGOs. Because many of the resources that sustain the local community come from outside through the governmental or NGO channels, the RO leaders' strategic positioning vis-à-vis those channels is critical for their organisational efforts in terms of both the resource flow and enhanced legitimacy. Not surprisingly, then, a privileged access to these sources of money and authority by some religious leaders engenders resentment, even if usually tacit, on the part of RO leaders who lack such access.

Religious organisations in HIV prevention

The RO-based HIV prevention activities illustrate how ideology is negotiated and deployed to enhance organisational identity and cohesion. Because HIV prevention education aims at raising awareness rather than building skills, it comes easily to religious leaders, sophisticated and passionate orators. Only minimal knowledge about HIV transmission and its consequences is necessary to teach others about the *need* to prevent infection. Not surprisingly, HIV prevention messages are frequently heard in congregations. Thus 81% of leaders interviewed in the institutional survey stated that they had talked about at least one form of HIV prevention during their congregations' main services in the several months preceding the survey and this percentage did not vary across denominational groups. The share of respondents in the women's survey who said that they had heard their congregation leaders talk about prevention during main services was only slightly lower – 75%.

Most religious leaders readily subscribe to well-established moralist clichés about premarital chastity and marital fidelity. Most are tolerant of condom use: in fact, 68% of institutional survey respondents approved of condom use by unmarried couples and 52% by married couples (again, with little denominational variation). It appears from the focus groups and interviews with leaders that higher ideological motives are rarely articulated and followed; local leaders, especially in rural areas, are typically unaware of or indifferent to the official pronouncements of their ROs' national leaders on matters of HIV prevention. This is not to say that at least some church leaders and most educated congregation members are incognisant of the frequent incongruence between religious and secular interpretations of HIV. As one interviewed teacher, who was also an active attendee of his church said, 'For us as religious people, this disease is a punishment for the infractions that we committed before God. Scientifically, I know that it is not true, but I am a religious person'.

Yet the common quandaries of a higher-order discourse – such as whether condoms should be allowed and even encouraged as a form of prevention – rarely take centre stage at the local level. Practical concerns about the church members' individual health and the congregation's collective well-being typically trump the directives received from the higher-ups, even in the Catholic Church, whose national leaders, echoing the Vatican, have voiced adamant opposition to condom use. Here is how a man from a rural Catholic parish explained the choice made by fellow parishioners despite the initial resistance of the parish priest:

> We agree that abstinence [from non-marital sex] is advantageous but the big defence is the condom, because among young people and adults alike one partner can easily cheat on the other… It was very difficult to talk about [condoms] in our parish because it was seen as promoting prostitution, but now we have proven that all we do is protect our lives, and even the priest has now talked about both in and outside the church about precautions to take against AIDS.

In churches where condom use is less controversial, the advice to use condoms with extramarital partners is often routinely explicit, as a Zionist man told us: 'On the days of prayer, when we leave [the church] around 6 pm, they tell us not to forget condoms when we go out to play'.

Reconciling church ideology with the secular message becomes easier as this message itself evolves. Thus in the case of Mozambique, a transition has taken place from a condom-focused campaign exemplified by the slogan '*Pensa direito, usa Jeito*' (Portuguese for: 'Think straight, use condom') to '*Andar fora é manyingui arriscado*' ('Fooling around is very risky'), an emphasis with which most church leaders can comfortably agree. Yet the effectiveness of the church formal prevention message, if such is ever articulated, is conditioned not so much by these semantic and vernacular nuances as by the social demographics of its audience. First, the overwhelming majority of church attendees are married women, who typically have no non-marital partners and who in general have little control over their sexual lives. The collective experience of listening to a pastor may heighten their awareness of HIV but the patriarchal norms of unquestionable submission to their husbands' will, typically reinforced in the church, do little to help translate this awareness into effective prevention. Furthermore, the prevention message, as it is usually framed and articulated by church leaders, is misleading as it equates women's propensity toward extramarital sex to that of men.

Unmarried adolescents are a demographic group that potentially stands to benefit from continuing HIV prevention exhortations. Church youth, however, may be a self-selected segment of that group, already with reduced predisposition to early sexual debut and to careless sexual practices. Besides, the dull repetitive rounds on staying chaste and using a condom if chastity becomes impossible can hardly ignite genuine interest among many young people.

Married men under the age of 40, the demographic group that perhaps is most prone to prolonged concurrent sexual partnering, i.e., the sexual behaviour that carries greatest risks, may not be adequately exposed to the church prevention message and to whatever sanctions that non-compliance with this message might trigger. These men rarely show up in church as many of them work outside the community and are simply too busy or too indifferent to attend church services and other events. Yet, membership of these men is critical to ROs' organisational strength. The RO leaders are particularly keen on attracting and retaining wealthier male church members because their membership promises significant financial inputs. To attract and keep the favours of such men, religious leaders often turn a blind eye on their conspicuous defiance of key religious moral teachings such as those pertaining to alcohol use, polygamy and casual extramarital sex. In the context of southern Mozambique, this rural economic elite is made up largely of current or recent labour migrants who have become relatively well-off from working in neighbouring South Africa. Having the means to pay the ever-rising bridewealth tab, migrants are disproportionately more likely to be polygynous; although most Christian churches officially reject polygyny, wealthy migrants are rarely reproved for having multiple wives. Likewise, while it is widely believed that migrants and other wealthy men tend to have casual sexual partners and that those partnerships are responsible for the spread of HIV in the community, RO leaders are generally reluctant to reprimand offenders for fear of losing the men's financial support and even their desertion to more accommodating ROs.[1]

Whereas prevention messages articulated by church leaderships may be too rare and too abstract for its audience to tune into, much of the HIV prevention-related discussions are carried out without a direct sanction and even without knowledge of the congregation top leaders. These discussions are most likely to happen in church youth groups and, especially, in church women's groups.[2] Thus, HIV-related conversations can emerge at women's group meetings, typically held on Thursdays in most churches, at which male church leaders are rarely present. A woman from a mainline Protestant church recounted how it happens at her congregation:

> At our Thursday meetings, we teach people to prevent AIDS. We teach that for a married couple to have unprotected sex, the two must be faithful to each other. Otherwise, they shouldn't [have unprotected sex]... We teach people that if they don't trust each other, they should get tested... We also teach about female condoms, and that a woman can very well carry a male condom, so that she gives it to her partner at the time of sexual intercourse.

In another mainline Protestant church, as a female member told us, the situation was not much different as prevention matters are discussed by church volunteers once a month, and the church pastor is only called upon to adjudicate between divergent opinions:

> We tell people that they should prevent this disease that does not yet have a cure. We explain that if someone has an extra-marital partner, they should use condoms when they have sexual relations... At the end of each month, we get together at 15 o'clock at the church. We pray first and then we talk, and everyone says what they know. And if we don't reach consensus on an issue, we take it to the pastor, and he says what's right and what's wrong.

When asked to elaborate on the content of those conversations, she added:

> In the group, we talk about women who don't trust their husbands and how to explain to them that they should use condoms. But some husbands do not accept using condoms and question the motives [behind their wives' suggestions] to use them. And from that point, we talk about what to do to get husbands to accept condom use.

Notably, because the church social space is highly gendered and church women's meetings never overlap with those of men (in congregations where men's meetings take place at all), these conversations rarely become the subject of cross-gender exchanges (Agadjanian and Menjívar 2008). For example, when asked about whether the same topics were raised at men's meetings, the woman just quoted could not come up with an answer: 'You should ask their [men's] counsellors', she replied. And even without men's physical presence, women's group discussions are imbued with the same patriarchal ideology that places women firmly into a subservient position relative to their husbands in general and instils acquiescence to husbands' sexual choices, in particular.

Although church-based prevention discourse on sexual practices, whether centralised or semi-autonomous, is often redundantly impracticable, confusing and misdirected, the HIV prevention rhetoric may serve as a powerful tool of institutional mobilisation because it provides an organisational purpose around which church members, especially church women, can rally, and which can further enhance their sense of belonging and therefore the church's strength and vitality. Involvement in HIV prevention activities also gives church leaders an opportunity to connect with secular authorities. Collaboration with state prevention campaigns, whatever their content and ideological colouring, helps enhance the status and legitimacy of the church in the eyes of both own church members and the leaders and members of other churches. At the same time, this collaboration does not directly jeopardise inter-church relations as church prevention efforts rarely cross congregational boundaries.

The organisational benefits of church HIV prevention discourse create incentives for church leaders to continue this discourse indefinitely. The RO-based prevention education thus shares the same irony that plagues its secular counterpart: in order to go on it must be perceived as ineffective. This paradoxical state of mind is arrived at through two main assumptions. First, not unlike the secular prevention messages, church-based prevention efforts assume that people are chronically under-informed about the risks of HIV/AIDS or that they choose to act foolishly and dangerously despite receiving exhaustively clear behavioural guidelines. In both cases, individual choices and agency are seen as central to the success of prevention education while structural constraints that influence and circumscribe individual behaviour are typically ignored or downplayed.

Second, even when church members receive abundant and forceful instructions that they can understand, they are seen as incapable of executing them once they step into the sinful world outside the congregation walls. An interviewed man expressed his view: 'We talk at church about [prevention], but at school, in the market people undo what they hear [in church]'. Yet even the message of prevention within the church when spread peer-to-peer is often not heeded – perhaps precisely because it is articulated by people who have no greater authority than any other of their church peers. Another interviewee put it this way:

> Ah, there is a saying 'a prophet is not honoured in his own land', which [in this case] means that if we who are from the same church teach each other, people ask themselves: 'what does he know that he's talking about it'. But if it's someone they don't know, they, I believe, will take notice.

The apparent failure of prevention efforts creates a sense of hopelessness. 'We are dying, we are asking to please give us a solution', said one participant, 'The condom doesn't work anymore, we are tired ... even Adam and Eve sinned because that thing is so sweet, so how can we leave sweet things to rot?' Her words were echoed by another interviewee: 'We all say the same ... just lament that God has given up to the evil, that Satan has more power than God. We ask every day, but God doesn't hear us, but Satan, for whom no one prays, has got more strength'.

Satan is powerful, and neither faithfulness nor condoms can stand up to him. Divine intervention becomes the only plausible hope, and the church prevention message thus morphs into one praising god and denouncing the devil. A male focus group participant thus summarised where he puts his trust:

> I want to ask my religious brothers to pray a lot in God's name, so that like the people of Israel we will be redeemed. On the day He decides He will eliminate this disease, like it happened with this last war [Mozambique's civil war, 1978–1992] that ended abruptly. That's why I want to beg them so that we continue to pray hard, ask our pastors to let us pray for this cause at the end of the service to end this [evil] that scientists cannot defeat and thus to show His power over us who praise Him.

Continuing collective praying, which shifts both the liabilities and the hopes surrounding the infection away from individual and societal actors into the realm of the divine, may diffuse the focus and the force of the prevention message but at the same time, serves as a powerful stimulant for congregation loyalism.

This is not to say that church-based prevention efforts cannot yield the intended benefits. Thus, one important area where these efforts can be truly effective is in encouraging people to get tested. This encouragement, however, benefits primarily young church members who consider marriage. Yet, for the majority of active church members – married women – this encouragement is of little use as a growing share of them undergo de facto mandatory HIV testing at antenatal consultations. And again, because married men's attendance of church services and of men's group meetings is so limited, many men simply do not hear this encouragement.

Perhaps the most notable (and often overlooked) contribution of RO-based teachings to HIV prevention is not in instilling righteous sexual attitudes and guiding corresponding behaviour but in advising church members to avoid contact with unclean cutting and piercing objects, especially those used in traditional healing practices. Thirty-eight per cent of the women's survey respondents said that their congregation leaders had offered this advice during main services. This advice is the least controversial ideologically and is fully congruent with the secular prevention message (even though the secular message, fixated on sexual transmission, has pushed the matter to the margins of HIV prevention). Once again, however, the real enemy of the church is not the infected razor blade used by a witchdoctor but the witchdoctor herself, a competitor to many churches, especially of the Pentecostal bend, in the healing business and a threat to church members' ideological devotion to the church and therefore to the church's organisational and ultimately financial health.

Religious organisations and HIV/AIDS-related assistance

Forty-five per cent of women's survey respondents indicated that they heard their leaders say during main services that congregation members should help AIDS patients. Yet the survey data also point to very limited involvement of ROs in the provision of assistance specifically targeted at AIDS-affected individuals and families. When asked whether they knew if their congregations had offered any sort of assistance to persons with AIDS or illnesses that looked like AIDS in the 12 months preceding the survey, only 10% of respondents answered affirmatively and only 3% knew that such assistance had been provided to more than two people.

Several factors may hamper ROs' active and effective involvement in the provision of care and support to HIV/AIDS-affected individuals and families. Some of these barriers are universal and are inherent to any community-level efforts to provide HIV/AIDS-related assistance. Thus congregation-based involvement in assistance to HIV-infected individuals is hindered by the still widespread stigma and fear of disclosure of a positive diagnosis. Although religious congregations are often said to be in a better position than other community organisations or state agencies to deal with these issues by gaining people's trust, no clear support for this argument has emerged from our data. As one Zionist woman noted: 'When someone has this disease, they don't want to know anything, they don't want to be visited [by church volunteers] because they think that those people after the visit will spread the news [of their disease] in the streets'. Of course, church volunteers do routinely reach out to sick congregation members and their families and survivors regardless of the nature and manifestation of their ailments. However, because HIV diagnosis is either unknown or undisclosed, HIV/AIDS-specific assistance such as encouraging antiretroviral therapy initiation and adherence cannot be offered.

ROs' ability to provide targeted care to their HIV-infected adherents is hampered not only by the lack of diagnosis, lingering stigma and fear of disclosure of HIV status, but also by a cloudy understanding of HIV-related opportunistic infections and their symptoms. Connections that some churches have with the health sector through their members facilitate church volunteers' education about these matters. In this regard, mainline churches hold an advantage over smaller, Pentecostal or Apostolic congregations as they are more likely to have nurses and even physicians among their members (Agadjanian and Menjívar 2008). In particular, district rural and semi-rural congregations' ties with city congregations of their denominations prove beneficial to the former. For example, a man from a mainline Protestant church told us about a physician member of the church, 'Dr. Komba [a pseudonym] who lives in Maputo. Sometimes we invite him here. Last year we invited him twice to give talks about AIDS and about other diseases like breast cancer'.

Any connection with a governmental institution or official is valued in the church as it adds to the church's legitimacy in general and to the reputation of the church leader in particular. As one woman put it, 'Church and government go together. Nothing is done in the church without government's knowledge. Everything should be reported to the government'. 'We can't do anything in the church', confirmed another woman, 'without informing the government'. Sometimes, local government officials may directly coax church leaders into HIV/AIDS-assistance activities such as praying for the sick in the community, providing home care or attending funerals. However, our data suggest that such requests are infrequent and are typically made through personal connections. Leaders of urban congregations, in particular those of mainline urban churches, are most likely to have strong personal ties in the government and in the large international NGOs that occasionally sponsor community-based assistance and care activities. As in the case of prevention-focused activities, larger urban congregations are also attractive to donors because of easy access, economy of scale and their leaders' relatively good literacy skills. Local RO-based NGOs that are established through such funding are then typically limited to a handful of well-connected urban-based churches whose leaders get along well, setting aside their ideological and organisational disagreements and personal animosities at least for the time when the money is flowing. As with many top-down community-based programs, these NGOs are poorly managed and their activities are grossly inefficient, with little systematic planning, haphazard selection of assistance targets and obscure accounting. Also importantly, the exclusive nature of these NGOs generates suspicions and even resentment on the part of the religious leaders who for one or another reason are left out.

Bottom-up cross-denominational collaborative initiatives, on the other hand, are crippled by a lack of financial resources, but perhaps even more so by the pervasive distrust among religious leaders who often deride one another as not truly Christian and readily suspect proselytising intentions in any attempts by their peers-competitors to step outside of the clearly drawn and carefully monitored member-ship boundaries. 'It's very difficult to get pastors from Zionist, Catholic, and other churches together in one place [i.e., to work together] because they think that other pastors want to grab their believers', said one male informant. Even when leaders of different churches get together and discuss, among other topics, AIDS-related matters, these meetings rarely lead to joint actions, especially those involving provision of support to sick members of other churches. 'Sometimes all of us [from different churches] meet to say prayers regarding this disease', commented an interviewed woman, 'Now, as far as visiting [the sick] and other such things, those have never happened. Each church takes care of its sick'.

To be sure, church leaders are usually quite adept at navigating the organisational boundaries and overt confrontations are extremely rare (and are emphatically denied by most church leaders during interviews). Yet, simmering tensions occasionally erupt into outright clashes and health, healing, death and burial, more than other issues or events, seem to trigger such eruptions. The following story told by a woman from a mainline Protestant congregation offers an illustration:

> There was a person in my church who had that disease [AIDS] but did not tell us about it. He left our church and went to a Zionist church to see if he gets better, but he ended up dead for he refused to accept that AIDS kills... On the day of his funeral we went there to sing our chants, but we were prohibited by that Zionist church who alleged that only they had the right to do it because the deceased had belonged to them.

While centrally orchestrated and deployed, church HIV/AIDS-assistance is fraught with risks of transgressing organisational borders and therefore may be resisted by distrustful competitors. Such assistance, when delivered as largely informal, minimally coordinated and by the low-key efforts of church rank-and-file members, especially women, may not elicit similar reactions simply because these efforts may not be construed by outsiders as church-organised undertakings. These activities normally revolve around home-based personal and household care; specific targets for them are typically decided upon at church women's meetings and they are carried out individually or in small groups, usually on an irregular ad hoc basis. Importantly, in most instances of such informal assistance, knowledge or suspicion of HIV diagnosis or HIV-related illness is not an explicit criterion for selecting or prioritising assistance targets.

Conclusion

The scale, vibrancy, and diversity of religious expressions in contemporary sub-Saharan Africa have reflected on many aspects of public life (Gifford 1998, Garner 2000b) and have long invited expectations that religion could be a major force in fighting the sub-continent's most dreadful scourge. However, the role of religion and ROs as effective agents of HIV/AIDS mitigation efforts has also been questioned. Research on the involvement of religion and religious organisations with HIV/AIDS has paid considerable heed to ideological and moral dilemmas shaping religious leaders' attitudes, pronouncements and actions. Issues surrounding condom use or stigma and discrimination have been at the centre of both scholarly and general public attention. Without discounting the significance of the ideological and moral discourse and the variation in how different denominations place emphases and accents in that discourse, our study has attempted to highlight other common factors that hinder the participation of ROs of all denominational banners in HIV prevention and care activities.

While many, if not most, religious leaders may be genuinely concerned about the health and well-being of the congregation members and other community residents, institutional pressures often overshadow these concerns. With a diminishing reservoir of unaffiliated individuals to satisfy the membership needs of a growing number of religious congregations and, accordingly, an ever exacerbating competition for new members, church organisational health becomes an increasingly important priority for many a religious leader. When an RO's organisational goals come into conflict with its ideological or moral codes, organisational goals may prevail. Political alliances – with government agencies and officials, powerful secular NGOs or with other ROs – are entered to ensure the church's organisational vigour thereby often further compromising its ideological and moral principles.

Ironically, while HIV prevention may be ideologically quite controversial, prevention activities, due to their low financial, organisational and logistical costs, yield a higher 'profit margin' in terms of organisational mobilisation and legitimacy than do care and support-related efforts. Not surprisingly then, prevention is greatly favoured by religious leaders. Emotionally charged yet devoid of personalised and concrete substance, the incessant prevention message is easy to articulate and to carry on indefinitely. This message helps galvanise church loyalty and mobilise members around a common perennial goal. At the same time, it is harmless for the church's relationships with the State, NGOs and other churches. In contrast, HIV/AIDS-related assistance is costly, organisationally complex, and because it targets concrete individuals who may or may not be part of the church, it may generate frictions and even overt clashes with other churches. In matters of HIV/AIDS care and support, religious leaders are then faced with an uneasy dilemma: on the one hand, individual congregations are usually too small numerically and weak financially to actively engage in effective HIV/AIDS-focused assistance. On the other hand, however, any attempt to achieve an economy of scale and to ensure effective provision of support to HIV/AIDS-affected persons beyond the congregation limits entails a potential for inter-church conflict.

It was not our intention to perform a formal assessment of success (or failure) of ROs' role in mitigating the impact of the HIV/AIDS epidemic in southern Mozambique. We should stress, however, that the constraints and contingencies identified and examined in our study, while hindering ROs' engagement in the fight against HIV/AIDS, do not prevent this engagement. In fact, ROs remain perhaps the most prominent community organisations that provide critically needed services to individuals and families affected by HIV/AIDS, especially in rural areas, where secular community organisations are ineffective or non-existent. As Garcia and Parker (2011) recently showed for Brazil, ROs can overcome their ideological and organisational differences and forge alliances to leverage resources and to deploy effective interventions among the population segments most affected by the HIV/AIDS epidemic. Although developing a recipe for a similar success in a setting like rural southern Mozambique is beyond the scope of this article, we believe that the path to success lies not only through building consensus and cooperation among ROs' leaders but even more so through harnessing the loosely organised yet tireless labour of ROs' volunteers, especially women for whom, as Agadjanian and Menjívar (2008) and Igreja and Lambranca (2009) showed, the church offers an unparalleled venue for social interaction, peer solidarity, spiritual and emotional self-fulfilment and community service.

Acknowledgements

The support of the Eunice Kennedy Shriver National Institute of Child Health and Human Development (*NICHD*) grant #R01HD050175 is gratefully acknowledged. Earlier versions of this paper were presented at the Conference on Religious Responses to HIV and AIDS, Columbia University, New York, 12–14 July 2010, and at the 18th International AIDS Conference, Vienna, Austria, 18–23 July 2010.

Notes

1. Although Pentecostal leaders are typically more insistent on compliance with church behavioural and moral guidelines than are leaders of other churches, we did not come across any sanctions applied against offenders comparable to those reported elsewhere (Garner 2000a, Parsitau 2009).
2. Women's groups typically include married or widowed/divorced women with marital and reproductive experience. In some churches, younger married women with few children (designated in the church lexicon with the Portuguese word *activistas,* or 'activists') hold separate meetings from those of older women. Younger, unmarried women usually attend youth groups' meeting.

References

Agadjanian, V. and Menjívar, C., 2008. Talking about the 'epidemic of the millennium': religion, informal communication, and HIV/AIDS in sub-Saharan Africa. *Social Problems,* 55 (3), 301–321.

Agadjanian, V. and Sen, S., 2007. Promises and challenges of faith-based AIDS care and support in Mozambique. *American Journal of Public Health,* 97 (2), 362–366.

Bate, S.C., ed., 2003. *Responsibility in a time of AIDS: a pastoral response by Catholic theologians and AIDS activists in Southern Africa.* South Africa: Cluster Publications.

Becker, F. and Geissler, P.W., eds., 2009. *AIDS and religious practice in Africa.* Leiden, The Netherlands: Brill NV.

Byamugisha, G., Steinitz, L.Y., Williams, G., and Zondi, P., 2002. *Journeys of faith: church-based responses to HIV and AIDS in three Southern African countries.* St. Albans, UK: TALC.

Casale, M., Nixon, S., Flicker, S., Rubincam, C., and Jenney, A., 2010. Dilemmas and tensions facing a faith-based organisation promoting HIV prevention among young people in South Africa. *African Journal of AIDS Research,* 9, 135–145.

Chitando, E., 2010. Sacred struggles: the World Council of Churches and the HIV epidemic in Africa. *In*: B. Bompani and M. Frahm-Arp, eds. *Development and politics from below: exploring religious spaces in the African state.* Basingstoke: Palgrave Macmillan, 218–239.

Francis, S.A. and Liverpool, J., 2009. A review of faith-based HIV prevention programs. *Journal of Religion and Health,* 48, 6–15.

Garcia, J. and Parker, R.G., 2011. Resource mobilization for health advocacy: Afro-Brazilian religious organizations and HIV prevention and control. *Social Science & Medicine,* 72 (12), 1930–1938.

Garner, R., 2000a. Safe sects? Dynamic religion and AIDS in South Africa. *Journal of Modern African Studies,* 38, 41–69.

Garner, R., 2000b. Religion as a source of social change in the new South Africa. *Journal of Religion in Africa,* 30, 310–343.

Gifford, P., 2010. *African Christianity: its public role.* Bloomington. IN: Indiana University Press.

Haddad, B., Olivier, J., and De Gruchy, S., 2008. *The potential and perils of partnership: Christian religious entities and collaborative stakeholders responding to HIV and AIDS in Kenya, Malawi and the DRC* [online]. Interim report. Cape Town and Scottsville, South Africa: ARHAP. Available from: http://www.arhap.uct.ac.za/downloads/TFUNAIDS_full_June2008.pdf [Accessed 15 June 2011].

Igreja, V. and Lambranca, B.D., 2009. The Thursdays as they live: Christian religious transformation and gender relations in postwar Gorongosa, Central Mozambique. *Journal of Religion in Africa*, 39 (3), 262–294.

Keikelame, M.J., Murphy, C.K., Ringheim, K.E., and Woldehanna, S., 2010. Perceptions of HIV/AIDS leaders about faith-based organisations' influence on HIV/AIDS stigma in South Africa. *African Journal of AIDS Research*, 9 (1), 63–70.

Krakauer, M. and Newbery, J., 2007. Churches' responses to HIV/AIDS in two South African communities. *Journal of the International Association of Physicians in AIDS Care*, 6 (1), 27–35.

Maman, S., Cathcart, R., Burkhardt, G., Ombac, S., and Behets, F., 2009. The role of religion in HIV-positive women's disclosure experiences and coping strategies in Kinshasa, Democratic Republic of Congo. *Social Science and Medicine*, 68, 965–970.

Mbilinyi, M. and Kaihula, N., 2000. Sinners and outsiders: the drama of AIDS in Rungwe. *In:* C. Baylies and J. Bujra, eds. *AIDS, sexuality and gender in Africa: collective strategies and struggles in Tanzania and Zambia*. London: Routledge, 75–95.

Ministry of Health, 2010. *Inquérito nacional de prevalência, riscos comportamentais e informação sobre o HIV e SIDA (INSIDA), 2009. Relatório final* [National Survey of HIV/AIDS prevalence, behavioural risks, and information, 2009: Final report]. Maputo, Mozambique: Ministry of Health of Mozambique.

Olivier, J., Cohrane, J.R., and Schmid, B., 2006. *APHAP literature review: working in a bounded field of unknowing* [online]. Cape Town: African Religious Health Assets Programme. Available from: http://www.arhap.uct.ac.za/downloads/arhaplitreview_oct2006. pdf [Accessed 15 June 2011].

Parsitau, D.S., 2009. 'Keep holy distance and abstain till He comes': interrogating a Pentecostal church's engagement with HIV/AIDS in the youth in Kenya. *Africa Today*, 56, 45–65.

Pfeiffer, J., 2004. Condom social marketing, Pentecostalism, and structural adjustment in Mozambique: a clash of AIDS prevention messages. *Medical Anthropology Quarterly*, 218, 77–103.

Regnerus, M.D. and Salinas, V., 2007. Religious affiliation and AIDS-based discrimination in sub-Saharan Africa. *Review of Religious Research*, 48 (4), 385–401.

Tiendrebeogo, G. and Bukyx, M., 2004. *Faith-based organisations and HIV/AIDS prevention and impact mitigation in Africa*. Amsterdam, The Netherlands: KIT Publishers.

Trinitapoli, J., 2006. Religious responses to AIDS in sub-Saharan Africa: an examination of religious congregations in rural Malawi. *Review of Religious Research*, 47 (3), 253–270.

Trinitapoli, J., 2009. Religious teachings and influences on the ABCs of HIV prevention in Malawi. *Social Science and Medicine*, 69, 199–209.

Trinitapoli, J. and Regnerus, M.D., 2006. Religion and HIV risk behaviours among married men: initial results from a study in rural sub-Saharan Africa. *Journal for the Scientific Study of Religion*, 45 (4), 505–528.

Watt, M.H., Maman, S., Jacobson, M., Laiser, J., and John, M., 2009. Missed opportunities for religious organizations to support people living with HIV/AIDS: findings from Tanzania. *AIDS Patient Care and STDs*, 23 (5), 389–394.

Zou, J., Yamanaka, Y., John, M., Watt, M., Ostermann, J., and Thielman, N., 2009. Religion and HIV in Tanzania: influence of religious beliefs on HIV stigma, disclosure, and treatment attitudes. *BMC Public Health*, 9, 75–87.

Pentecostalism and AIDS treatment in Mozambique: Creating new approaches to HIV prevention through anti-retroviral therapy

James Pfeiffer

Department of Global Health/Department of Health Services, School of Public Health, University of Washington, Seattle, USA

Pentecostal fervor has rapidly spread throughout central and southern Mozambique since the end of its protracted civil war in the early 1990s. In the peri-urban bairros and septic fringes of Mozambican cities African Independent Churches (AICs) with Pentecostal roots and mainstream Pentecostals can now claim over half the population as adherents. Over this same period another important phenomenon has coincided with this church expansion: the AIDS epidemic. Pentecostalism and HIV have travelled along similar vectors and been propelled by deepening inequality. Recognising this relationship has important implications for HIV/AIDS prevention and treatment strategies. The striking overlap between high HIV prevalence in peri-urban populations and high Pentecostal participation suggests that creative strategies, to include these movements in HIV/AIDS programming, may influence the long-term success of HIV care and the scale-up of anti-retroviral treatment (ART) across the region. The provision of ART has opened up new possibilities for engaging with local communities, especially Pentecostals and AICS, who are witnessing the immediate benefits of ARV therapy. Expanded treatment may be the key to successful prevention as advocates of a comprehensive approach to the epidemic have long argued.

Introduction

Pentecostal fervor has rapidly spread throughout central and southern Mozambique since the end of its protracted civil war in the early 1990s. In the peri-urban bairros and septic fringes of Mozambican cities African Independent Churches (AICs) with Pentecostal roots and mainstream Pentecostals can now claim over half the population as adherents (see Figure 1, INE 1999). Over this same period another important phenomenon has coincided with this church expansion: the AIDS epidemic. In urban areas of Sofala and Manica Province, current HIV prevalence among adults is estimated at nearly 20% (Ministry of Health 2009). Prevalence in Maputo to the South has surged even higher. Currently in Mozambique, HIV prevalence is highest in precisely the same communities where Pentecostals and AICs have the most adherents.

While casual observers speculate that the churches have perhaps become popular in response to the social suffering and mortality produced by AIDS, the Pentecostal

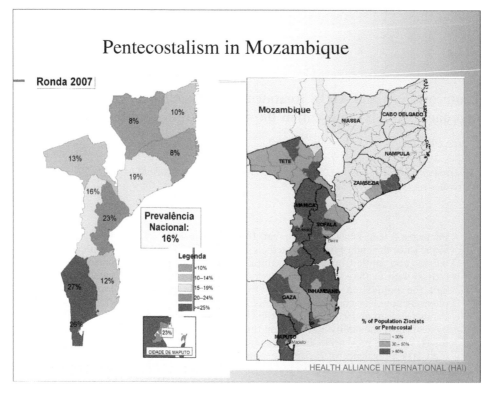

Figure 1. Pentecostalism and HIV in Mozambique.

movement had already gained momentum in the mid-1990s before local communities were recognising and experiencing the epidemic. However, it is argued here that the simultaneous emergence of the two phenomena in Mozambique was not coincidental. Pentecostalism and HIV have travelled along similar vectors and have been propelled by the same recent socio-economic and political transformations. Recognising this relationship has important implications for HIV/AIDS prevention and treatment strategies.

HIV prevalence is higher in the centre and south of the country because of proximity to Zimbabwe and South Africa where rates rose to alarming levels much earlier. Male labour migration to South African mines, especially from Mozambique's southern provinces, has likely contributed to the increase in HIV prevalence. Similarly, Pentecostals and AICs already had large followings in South Africa and Zimbabwe by the 1990s with their pastors and evangelists eagerly awaiting opportunities to spread their message to Mozambique. At the end of the war, borders opened, traffic increased, and populations moved back and forth more freely; HIV prevalence in Mozambique rose steadily and rapidly. These same circumstances allowed Pentecostal preachers and proselytisers from Mozambique's neighbours to establish new churches and train local pastors from communities eager to hear their healing message. HIV and the Pentecostal messages travelled the same roads into Mozambique.

Inequality, HIV and church growth

However, beyond the opening of borders and increased movement between countries, other important transformations were under way in Mozambique that have fostered both the spread of HIV and the popularity of the Pentecostal message. After its experiment with socialism in the post-independence period, Mozambique was pressed by the World Bank and IMF to adopt a structural adjustment programme (SAP) in the late 1980s, and by the 1990s the economic reforms began to have a widespread effect. The impact of the SAP on public sector services is familiar: social services were cut back, fees for services introduced, civil servant salaries lowered, social safety nets eliminated and productive resources privatised (Marshall 1990, Cliff 1991, Hanlon 1996, Pfeiffer 2002, Rowden 2009). In Mozambique, women's cooperatives were dismantled, state-led purchase of rural produce from women producers ended and subsidised food prices for the poor were eliminated (Pitcher 2002).

By the end of the 1990s, Mozambique's economy was growing at an annual 7–8%, and has been heralded as a beacon of economic progress in Africa; one of the World Bank's few examples of economic recovery after the implementation of structural adjustment on the continent. But the benefits of this growth have not trickled down (Fauvet 2000). The recent national Rural Income Survey (2008) reveals that from 2002 to 2008 incomes have remained flat or declined for the great majority of the population while elites have accumulated larger and larger portions of the national wealth. Mean total income increased while median total income declined. The total income of the richest 10% is 44 times that of the poorest 10%, up from 23 times in 2002 and 35 times in 2005. Recent national nutritional data reveal that malnutrition rates remained unchanged since the war, and in some areas have worsened, providing further evidence that the poor have not shared in the new wealth (Ministry of Health 2005, Hanlon and Smart 2008). Corruption and accumulation have reached new heights in the capital among the well-placed. It is argued here that this rapidly steepening social gradient may have fostered both the expansion of churches and the transmission of HIV.

Increased social inequality and economic vulnerability, especially among women, has become the familiar hallmark and legacy of structural adjustment across Africa. As Peter Piot, former Executive Director of UNAIDS, has stated, 'Structural adjustment raises particular problems for governments because most of the factors which fuel the AIDS pandemic are also those factors that seem to come into play in structural adjustment programs' (cited in Poku 2002, p. 538). Growing inequality and declining social services have pushed many women into survival sex work and Mozambicans speak openly and candidly about the perceived rapid expansion of transactional sex (usually referred to as *prostituição*, or prostitution, in interviews) in their country since the end of the war (Pfeiffer 2004, Pfeiffer *et al.* 2007).

As the growth in inequality, economic insecurity, withdrawal of the state and declines in public services may have helped propel the AIDS epidemic, these same social transformations led many, especially women, to Pentecostal and Zionist churches in search of spiritual healing, mutual aid and refuge: refuge from accusations of 'prostitution' (the term used by women respondents) and abusive husbands, and refuge for women with no money in a social world in which access to cash is increasingly critical to survival (Pfeiffer *et al.* 2007). Data from a survey conducted in Manica Province suggest that social and economic inequality indexes the variegated religious landscape where Christian faith affiliations closely calibrate to social class (Pfeiffer *et al.* 2007). Zionists and other AICs are the churches of the poorest, while more mainstream Pentecostals, such as the Assemblies of God and the *Reino de Deus* target the working class and aspiring professionals; the Catholic Church retains some influence in poor neighbourhoods but is dominated by middle classes and elites given its close historical association with the Portuguese colonial project. More mainline Protestant faiths are most popular among well-educated urban Mozambicans. The Protestant Christian Council of Mozambique (CCM) founded by Methodist, Anglicans and Presbyterians, barely recognises the existence of AICs or Pentecostals, yet the CCM remains the principal conduit between the state and protestant groupings while participating CCM faiths represent a very small percentage of the population.

The Mozambique experience mirrors that of Pentecostal movements around the world. As urban historian, Mike Davis, states, 'Since 1970, and largely because of its appeal to slum women and its reputation for being color-blind, it [Pentecostalism] has been growing into what is arguably the largest self-organised movement of urban poor people on the planet'. (Davis 2004, p. 32, see also Comaroff 1985, Cox 1995, Corten and Marshall-Fratani 2001, Meyer 2004). The striking overlap between high HIV prevalence peri-urban populations and high Pentecostal participation suggests that creative strategies to include these movements in HIV/AIDS programming may determine the long-term success of the HIV care and ART scale-up itself across the region.

Given the uncontroversial and easily recognisable observation that Pentecostals and AICs have grown remarkably quickly in the same areas hit hardest by AIDS, it might come as a surprise how little direct engagement there has been with these church movements by international NGOs, the Ministry of Health or aid agencies in combating AIDS. There is still little in the public health literature on Pentecostalism and HIV in Africa. While home-based care (HBC) programmes have often channeled resources into some Pentecostal church-based HBC organisations, the great majority of churches have been by-passed, most notably the Zions. The Catholic Church participates at high levels in the national discussion on the epidemic but also does not link it with the Pentecostals.

There are a number of potential explanations for this gap: the legacy of state hostility to religion, the relatively little attention paid to HIV/AIDS in Mozambique in general or lack of resources to mount effective community outreach to churches. Another factor that inhibits engagement may be the negative preconception among foreign aid workers and planners about the nature and history of the churches. Many assume that the churches are products of US or Brazilian evangelists and funding and are not seen as legitimate civil society organisations by secular aid workers. International Christian NGOs may see them as competitors for the same terrain or denigrate their localised versions of Christianity, as earlier missionaries had.

However, I argue here that the failure to include or engage these dynamic movements is also, in part, the result of the same deepening inequalities that have helped produce the epidemic. The aid funding now streaming into Mozambique to support both prevention and treatment efforts is largely captured by emerging urban elites and shared with the expatriate NGO community that has ballooned in response to aid funding increases, especially in the capital city of Maputo. Inequality within the Christian community in Mozambique has been a barrier to Pentecostal and AIC inclusion as aid funding is channeled to mainstream churches. Public health and medical services are dominated by foreign aid workers and local elites who by and large do not belong to the new churches and view them with dismissiveness or great suspicion. In other words, the rapid increase in social inequality has generated parallel processes of institutional exclusion that impedes the response to the epidemic; it is difficult to define or identify a meaningful forum in Mozambique today in which these churches of the poor can be included in the national dialogue on HIV/AIDS.

Based on the author's ethnographic and survey data from central Mozambique, efforts at condom promotion through social marketing have been ineffective in part because the new church communities have not been solicited in any meaningful way to develop programmes or voice concerns (Pfeiffer 2004). Not surprisingly, given their history elsewhere, the AICs and Pentecostals tend to be anti-condom since they view them as promoting *'prostituição'*, or prostitution – a critical concern to them and their communities given the perceived rapid expansion of transactional sex in the region that reportedly ranges from full time sex work to occasional transactions to secure food and clothing (Pfeiffer *et al.* 2007). They have reacted strongly to the social marketing campaign and actively prohibit members from using condoms. Given that these churches claim over 50% membership in the city neighbourhoods with the highest HIV prevalence, this response should be viewed as alarming by the public health community. The potentially harmful and narrow focus on individual 'behaviour change', whether through condom social marketing or the ABC approach, neglects the more important and complex work of dialogue with Pentecostal and AIC communities to develop shared strategies to support poor communities and church members (Pfeiffer 2004). The limited focus on change in sexual behaviour and prevention may have in fact closed the possibility of dialogue with the church movements.

ART scale-up: treatment and prevention

To the extent that religious organisations have been enlisted to fight the AIDS epidemic, the emphasis has been on either prevention or provision of palliative care. However, in 2004, the public sector National Health System began providing anti-retroviral treatment (ART) for free to its citizens in sites throughout the country (Pfeiffer *et al.* 2010). The commitment to provide anti-retrovirals to everyone who needs them has shifted the framework for AIDS strategies in Mozambique. Rather than remaining locked in a stalemate about condoms versus abstinence, the provision of ART has opened up new possibilities for engaging with local communities, especially Pentecostals and AICs, who are witnessing the immediate benefits of ARV therapy. In contemporary Mozambique, expanded treatment may be the key to successful prevention, as advocates of a comprehensive approach to the epidemic have long argued.

An estimated 1.5 million Mozambicans are HIV-positive, and about 400,000 are eligible for ART. Funded by a consortium of donors, including PEPFAR, the World Bank, the Global Fund, the Clinton Foundation and others, treatment has been scaled up gradually; initially through a vertical day-hospital model and eventually through the integration of HIV care and treatment into hundreds of health units in the public primary health care system. By March 2010, 182,000 Mozambicans had initiated ART, over 45% of those eligible (Ministry of Health 2010). As infrastructure is established and thousands more get treatment each month, the urgent need for better community mobilisation has also become apparent. In the current phase, systemic problems are emerging that confirm the importance of social mobilisation for scale-up success. For example, in provinces where the author has worked, only about 35% of pregnant women who test HIV-positive in the prevention of maternal-to-child-transmission (pMTCT) sites follow up with the ART programme to get into the treatment system (Pfeiffer *et al.* 2010). There is a significant loss of more HIV-positive women even after they get registered for ART. Only a handful in some sites are actually managing to initiate ART as they drop out of the long series of preparatory visits. In some provinces, nearly 50% of those who test positive at separate VCT sites did not follow up (Pfeiffer *et al.* 2010). While adherence to ART appeared to be quite good at first, there are signs that adherence is beginning to falter in many sites across Mozambique (Ministry of Health 2010). There continue to be important challenges to educating and informing communities that testing and treatment services are available, and then explaining what the services are and how they work. Addressing all these challenges will involve engagement with key actors at the community-level to provide support.

The social context of the ART roll-out will shape its success, and the social consequences of offering treatment are profound. The overlap between high prevalence urban populations and high Pentecostal and AIC participation means that the success of creative strategies to include these movements, in all their variations, may influence the long-term success of the scale-up itself.

Churches and ART scale-up in two provinces: new research findings

In the two provinces where the author has worked with Health Alliance International (HAI), a US-based NGO, and the Mozambique Ministry of Health (MOH) in scaling up ART and PMTCT services, recent research on church influences on treatment follow-up indicates the extent to which the provision of ART has opened up church discourse on HIV and created the potential for collaboration with the health system to promote and support HIV testing and treatment. At present, in Manica and Sofala provinces, the relationship between the national health system and AIC and Pentecostal churches is minimal with virtually no structural linkages. HBC programmes organised by local civil society groups, with support from HAI and MOH, have connected with some local Pentecostal congregations, but these efforts still remain somewhat disconnected from the ART sites.

Data were collected at two urban sites around the major MOH ART clinics in the cities of Beira (Sofala Province) and Chimoio (Manica Province) from 2007 to 2009. The research, primarily qualitative and exploratory, sought to determine how membership in churches may influence how members choose to get tested for HIV and follow up with treatment. Research teams completed qualitative open-ended individual interviews with 78 adherent HIV-positive patients who were church members and 23 non-adherent patients (also church members). Snowball sampling was used to select adherent and non-adherent respondents through HIV-positive activists who worked with the health system to follow up with patients. (The recruitment approach was approved by both University of Washington and

Mozambique MOH ethical review boards.) Twenty church leaders, 13 health workers and 8 HIV/AIDS patient organisation activists were also interviewed. Three focus group discussions (FGDs) with adherent church members, five FGDs with HIV-positive patients or HBC group members and five FGDs with non-HIV-positive church members were completed. Research team members attended dozens of church services and events. Comprehensive maps of churches in the targeted neighborhoods were also completed.

As results are examined, initial findings provide a snapshot of both the vital influence of church membership on decisions to test and seek treatment, the changing discourse on HIV within churches that treatment availability has produced, and the ongoing sense of exclusion from public health initiatives that most churches and their members experience. Several key themes have emerged from the research findings. First, compared to earlier work conducted among churches in the area, there is now greater variation among pastors across the spectrum of Pentecostals and AICs in attitudes toward HIV/AIDS (Chapman *et al.* 1999, Pfeiffer 2004). In earlier research, in the early 2000s, virtually no pastor interviewed discussed HIV openly and the topic was still off limits in church services. By 2008, this recent research found a growing recognition and 'normalisation' of the epidemic. For example, one pastor at Igreja Pentecostal stated:

> To tell you the truth, there are many believers [church members] that are having problems with HIV/AIDS. So people are no longer judging. . .in various churches people have had problems and deaths, and its being seen now as something normal, its already seen as something normal.

Researchers for this project discovered that in some instances church members reported disclosing their HIV-positive status to their pastors rather than spouses, family members or friends. In several instances, pastors had disclosed their own HIV-positive status and treatment experience to their congregations. In a number of cases pastors were reportedly encouraging their members to get tested and to get into treatment. For example, one Zion Christian Church (ZCC) female member stated:

> They [pastors] ask people to get tested – not as an obligation but as a necessity for us all. They say that everyone has to do the test to know what is your status and to know early because if one knows one's status sooner, when you come to church with our prayers that person is more supported. They always say this now.

Another woman church member at Igreja Pentecostal remarked:

> [T]he Sunday before last I was in church and the pastor was saying that. . .when a person knows they have the HIV virus they have to go to the hospital and follow-up and start treatment, because there are many orphans since many people didn't want to go to the hospital earlier. He gave us this counseling. . .

Many churches, and not only those involved with externally supported HBC programmes, are already providing support to ill home-bound members. While this was common among churches previously, the apparent opening up of discussion on HIV has generated new levels of social and material support, at least among some congregations, for fellow members known to be HIV-positive.

The interviews among women revealed that active women's associations in many of the local churches have structures to disseminate information about testing and treatment and could potentially provide adherence assistance to HIV-positive women on ART. Maternal child health nurses interviewed during this research reported that some women coming in for antenatal visits (where they will get HIV testing and treatment referrals) are accompanied by members of church groups, and prayer sessions are conducted before and after the ANC visits. There were a number of reports of women giving birth in churches with support from church mid-wives (see also Chapman 2003). Loss-to-follow-up among poor pregnant HIV-positive women is emerging as one the major challenges to HIV care scale-up in Africa, and the special appeal of Pentecostal and AIC churches to this demographic group suggests an urgency to establish more direct engagement with them.

While the interviews indicate a growing openness within church discourse on HIV/AIDS produced by access to treatment services, evidence of a continued sense of exclusion was also apparent. None of the pastors not already involved in structured HBC programmes, reported having any contact with health system representatives or aid organisations concerning HIV/AIDS related issues or programmes. While a complete census of clinical health workers and religious affiliation was not completed for this research, dozens of health workers were contacted and over 90% identified themselves as Catholic, expressing little under-standing or awareness of the extent of Pentecostal and AIC influence in their patient populations. In other words, religious difference is institutionalised in the provision of health services themselves. Pentecostal church members were most likely to be found among lower level workers, if at all. There were no medical doctors in the two provinces who are also church members. The institutional religious divide has broad implications for service provision and community outreach efforts, and reflects the broader social inequality that has worsened since the end of the war.

Conclusions: bridging the gap between services and religious communities

Several important trends in Pentecostal and AIC church engagement with HIV/AIDS programmes and services are apparent in Mozambique. As organisations of the peri-urban poor and working class, the Pentecostals and AICs have captured the imagination of the same demographic that is ostensibly but inadequately targeted by the HIV/AIDS services industry. Church leaders express strong interest in engaging more directly with health care providers in addressing the epidemic, however, institutional barriers erected by growing social inequality, and its religious expres-sion, present major challenges to developing and implementing effective mobilisation programmes. Health education messaging for prevention has largely been ineffective in part because the churches have been left out or have turned away from messages deemed by them to be provocative or inappropriate.

The scale-up of ART has opened up new room for discussion about AIDS among many churches, as evidenced by pastors emboldened to disclose to their own congregations, and by church support mechanisms to help members follow up with treatment options. The availability of treatment, and the hope it has inspired, provides a new opportunity to reach out to religious communities to participate in testing and treatment support that provides direct and visible results for church members. In this sense the experience with the churches in Mozambique supports the argument for a comprehensive approach in which treatment and prevention are not represented as competing public health priorities. The provision of treatment in these religious communities appears to have provided a major shift in consciousness among leaders and lay members and provided grounds for a new social solidarity focused on the immediacy of saving lives; a project less complicated by the struggles over moral discourse and sexual behaviour. Overcoming the unwillingness to openly discuss HIV is the first crucial step toward prevention.

While the public national health system has been more effective than anticipated in scaling-up ART provision – exceeding the projections in the 2003 national plan – the growing struggles around loss-to-follow-up and adherence reveal the system's limits, unless it can become more agile and proactive in mobilising communities, especially religious constituencies. Barriers to progress in prevention and treatment in this next phase of the epidemic will not come from the churches or non-compliant Mozambican communities, but rather from the international aid community's inattention to the burgeoning Pentecostal and AIC movements. Many in the aid and public health world are wary of supporting the apparently conservative social vision of the Pentecostals and AICs, with their aversion to condom promotion and their promotion of a patriarchal theology. To be sure, the aid response to the church movements has been complicated by the ideologically driven restrictions around condom promotion and emphasis on abstinence messaging imposed during the Bush administration. Local NGO and MOH directors, planners, and managers also inhabit different social worlds and may not have recognised nor experienced the church dynamism and vitality in poor communities.

On the other hand, many Pentecostal pastors and women's groups within churches are eager to help care for their members with AIDS and advance the process of testing, referral and treatment. The Pentecostals and AICs should be seen as partners in this process not as obstacles. While the national Organisation of Mozambican Women (known locally as OMM), created after independence, still functions, there are few if any organised women's associations that can advocate for poor women to receive better access to better quality health services in the provinces. The churches may provide among the best openings to the vast poor communities, especially poor women of reproductive age, that the aid world seeks to treat in southern Africa, and as a result they may also offer the best new potential for effective prevention. Principled public health efforts can, instead, work with expanding church movements by helping their members understand the meaning of testing and treatment, and linking these organic community structures to public HIV/AIDS treatment services. Such an approach would not require an approval of their conservative social philosophy, substituting them for state services or endorsing their positions on condoms and sexual behaviour. As these churches become more deeply engaged in the struggle against AIDS, inevitably contradictions will emerge around the need for open discussion about sexuality amidst the conservative moral discourses of Pentecostalism, and the urgency to address gender HIV disparities within a patriarchal institutional environment. But these challenges are not unique to Pentecostalism; avoiding religious institutions in public health programming is not viable anywhere. However, because of these contradictions and sensitivities the initial effort in Mozambique should establish a shared goal of supporting members to initiate treatment, helping them to stay on treatment and creating community dialogue with the health system so that services can better meet community demands.

Through such partnership-building and dialogue, promotion of effective community-based prevention strategies becomes viable.

Importantly, this will require resistance to the ongoing conditionalities of structural adjustment so that donor support to the public sector national health system can be increased to guarantee that basic HIV/AIDS clinical care can be delivered effectively, and that the system itself can accommodate, embrace and respond to a more robust community mobilisation strategy (Rowden 2009). No HIV/AIDS treatment or prevention efforts can be successful or sustainable with the continued fiscal constraints on training and hiring of public sector health workers and the ongoing ceilings on infrastructure and recurrent expenditures. The churches have surged among those left behind in the shift to market fundamentalism and structural adjustment that have characterised the last two decades in Mozambique. They also provide a ready and willing ally in the struggle to bring services, if adequately funded, to those most marginalised and vulnerable.

Acknowledgements

The recent research described here was supported by a grant from the National Institute of Child Health and Development (NICHD). Health Alliance International provided additional logistical support for this project.

References

Chapman, R., 2003. Endangering safe motherhood in Mozambique: prenatal care as reproductive risk. *Social Science and Medicine*, 57 (2), 355–374.

Chapman, R., Davissone, P., Machobo, F., and Pfeiffer, J., 1999. *Community leadership and health: a rapid ethnographic study of three zones in Manica Province*. Chimoio, Mozambique: Mozambique Ministry of Health and Health Alliance International.

Cliff, J., 1991. The war on women in Mozambique: health consequences of South African destabilisation, economic crisis, and structural adjustment. *In*: M. Turshen, ed. *Women and health in Africa*. Trenton, NJ: Africa World Press, 15–33.

Comaroff, J., 1985. *Body of power, spirit of resistance*. Chicago: University of Chicago.

Corten, A. and Marshall-Fratani, R., eds., 2001. *Between babel and Pentecost: transnational Pentecostalism in Africa and Latin America*. Bloomington, IN: Indiana University Press.

Cox, H., 1995. *Fire from heaven: the rise of Pentecostal spirituality and the reshaping of religion in the twenty-first century*. Reading, MA: Addison-Wesley.

Davis, M., 2004. Planet of slums: Urban involution and the informal proletariat. *New Left Review*, 26, 5–34.

Fauvet, P., 2000. Mozambique: growth with poverty, a difficult transition from prolonged war to peace and development. *Africa Recovery*, 14, 3.

Hanlon, J., 1996. *Peace without profit: how the IMF blocks rebuilding in Mozambique*. Oxford: James Currey.

Hanlon, J. and Smart, E., 2008. *Do bicycles equal development in Mozambique?*. Oxford: James Currey.

INE (Instituto Nacional de Estatistica), 1999. *II Recenseamento Geral da Populacao e Habitacao, 1997* (Second General Census). Maputo: Government of Mozambique.

Marshall, J., 1990. Structural adjustment and social policy in Mozambique. *Review of African Political Economy*, 17 (48), 28–43.

Meyer, B., 2004. Christianity in Africa: from African independent to pentecostal-charismatic churches. *Annual Review of Anthropology*, 33, 447–474.

Ministry of Health, Mozambique, 2005. *National Nutrition Survey*. Maputo: Mozambique Ministry of Health.

Ministry of Health, Mozambique, 2009. *National HIV/AIDS Survey of prevalence, risks, behaviours and information (INSIDA)*. Maputo: Mozambique Ministry of Health.

Ministry of Health, Mozambique, 2010. *National medical assistance department (DNAM), routine report*. Maputo: Mozambique Ministry of Health.

Pfeiffer, J., 2002. African independent churches in Mozambique: healing the afflictions of inequality. *Medical Anthropology Quarterly*, 16 (2), 176–199.

Pfeiffer, J., 2004. Condom social marketing, pentecostalism, and structural adjustment in Mozambique: a clash of AIDS prevention messages. *Medical Anthropology Quarterly*, 18 (1), 77–103.

Pfeiffer, J., Montoya, P., Baptista, A., Karagianis, M., Pugas, M., Micek, M., Johnson, W., Sherr, K., Gimbel, S., Baird, S., Lambdin, B., and Gloyd, S., 2010. Integration of HIV/AIDS services into African primary health care: lessons learned for health system strengthening in Mozambique. *Journal of the International AIDS Society*, 13 (3), 1–9.

Pfeiffer, J., Sherr, K., and Augusto, O., 2007. The holy spirit in the household: Pentecostalism, gender, and neoliberalism in Mozambique. *American Anthropologist*, 109 (4), 688–700.

Pitcher, A.M., 2002. *Transforming Mozambique: the politics of privatization, 1975–2000*. Cambridge: Cambridge University Press.

Poku, N., 2002. Poverty, debt and Africa's HIV/AIDS crisis. *International Affairs*, 78 (3), 531–546.

Rowden, R., 2009. *The deadly ideas of neoliberalism: how the IMF has undermined public health and the fight against AIDS*. London: Zed Books.

Free love: A case study of church-run home-based caregivers in a high vulnerability setting

Robin Root[a] and Arnau van Wyngaard[b]

[a]Department of Sociology and Anthropology, Baruch College, The City University of New York, New York, NY, USA; [b]Shiselweni Reformed Church Home-based Care Organisation, Swaziland

The purpose of this study is to explore the concept of religious health assets (RHA) and its relevance to HIV/AIDS. This manuscript describes the experiences of caregivers with a church-run home-based care organisation in Swaziland, site of the world's highest HIV prevalence (42%). In light of reduced antiretroviral treatment rollout in some areas of Africa, strengthening mechanisms of treatment support with HIV prevention has never been more critical. One modality may be community home-based care (CHBC), a core feature of the World Bank's Multi-Country HIV/AIDS Program for Africa. Yet, these entities, and the frontline activities of local congregations, remain underexplored. Part of a larger anthropological study of religion and HIV/AIDS in Swaziland, this manuscript draws on 20 semi-structured caregiver interviews to discern patterns in motivations; perceived client needs; care practices; and meanings of religiosity. Thirteen participants were care coordinators who oversaw approximately 455 caregivers across nearly half of the 22 communities served. Grounded theory analysis suggested that caregivers facilitated vital decisions around HIV testing, HIV disclosure, treatment uptake/adherence, as well as reduced HIV stigma. Also salient was the importance of a Christian ethos, in the form of 'talk' and 'love', as critical culturally situated care practices. Having expanded to an estimated 600 caregivers and 2500 home-based clients between 2006 and 2009, participants' reports intimated their roles as agents of broader social transformation. This article contributes to the expanding study of RHA and challenges authoritative global public health strategies that have largely marginalised local religious aspects of HIV/AIDS. Future applied research examining how 'home' and 'church' may be vital public health settings outside of, but integral to, formal health services and HIV programming is warranted.

Introduction

'I told the man, "I have a plan [so you can tell your wife you're HIV positive]". I knew the husband and wife each was positive, and that the other didn't know. I told him I'd come to their home one Saturday with a slaughtered chicken and ask her to cook it with porridge . . . I visited and we all told stories. Then the man said, "Now, my wife, what if I told you I'm HIV positive?" She said, "I would just accept you as you are, because you are still a human being". I said, "This is your chance". So he said, "I am HIV positive". She said, "I'm also positive", and went to get her handbag. "You see this? I never, ever put it

down, because it has my tablets [antiretroviral therapy]". My heart was so sad, because the man had hidden his tablets under a tree outside the homestead. He dug a hole and everyday he'd go to the tree [to take the ART in secret].[1]
– Church-run home-based caregiver

Faced with the world's highest HIV prevalence rates, poor health care infrastructure and limited economic resources, hard-hit communities in many parts of Africa have mobilised to mitigate worsening conditions. Although these 'variables' are common across many resource-limited regions of the world, they are also culturally situated. This means that in places where religion is a salient feature of social life, investigation of the roles that religion, broadly conceived, may play in mediating multiple vulnerabilities is critical. In Swaziland, site of the study described here and the world's highest national population-based adult (25.9%, Central Statistical Office 2008) and antenatal (42%, UNAIDS 2009) HIV prevalence rates, there has been substantial growth in registered church organisations since the 1990s (Pan African Christian AIDS Network 2008). The country's institutional saturation by local congregations and their possible relevance to HIV/AIDS are indicated by the estimated one church per 183 Swazis (personal communication, B. Langa, July 2006) versus one HIV testing and counselling site (HTC) per 6180 (National Emergency Response Council on HIV/AIDS [NERCHA] 2010). To explore one aspect of this institutional efflorescence, the manuscript draws on focused ethnographic and formal qualitative data to explore the experiences of volunteer caregivers with a church-run home-based care organisation in Swaziland. More broadly, the article aims to identify whether and in what ways local religious modalities might mitigate HIV/AIDS in places where conventional public health resources cannot reach people's homes.

Investigation of religion and HIV/AIDS is important because to many health researchers and policy-makers, the idea of Christianity benefiting HIV/AIDS initiatives in Africa may seem unfamiliar or even uncomfortable. While concerns over religious obstacles to condom promotion are well-founded, to limit scholarly investigation of Christianity and HIV/AIDS to debates over abstinence, fidelity and condom campaigns (Allen and Heald 2004) may negate the deeply felt and institutionalised presence of Christianity (Meyer 2004, Gifford 2008) that affects millions of people living with HIV/AIDS (PLWHA) and their families in Africa on a daily basis (Agadjanian and Sen 2007, Becker and Geissler 2007). As a result, assumptions that religion inherently obstructs HIV/AIDS programming may have eclipsed opportunities to deliver HIV/AIDS services. In light of these politics, the article seeks to contribute to an emergent social scientific literature that examines the multifactorial significance of religion and HIV/AIDS (Cochrane 2006, Adogame 2007) in many parts of the world that challenges authoritative global public health strategies that have often marginalised and politicised religious aspects of HIV/AIDS. The African Religious Health Assets Programme (ARHAP), an international network of scholars and practitioners originating out of the University of Cape Town, has introduced the concept of religious health assets (RHA) to begin theorising the complex dynamics of religion and HIV/AIDS, primarily as a means of enhancing public health systems and community well-being (ARHAP 2006). In both respects, RHA provides the framing conceptual framework of this article.

Research setting

The Kingdom of Swaziland

Swaziland offers both the sociocultural and, tragically, the epidemiological context for exploring relationships between religion and HIV/AIDS. With the world's highest HIV prevalence, a 33% orphan rate, and an estimated 46-year life expectancy at birth (World Bank Group 2010), the social fabric of Swazi society is wrent in unprecedented ways. From one-room wattle and daub to expansive concrete structures, churches are ubiquitous features of the country's physical and social landscape, a terrain where Swazis say 'people are dying left and right'. In 2008, 22 facilities provided antiretroviral therapy (ART) (UNAIDS 2008). However, with only 15 physicians (NERCHA 2008) to treat the 190,000 children and adults (HIV InSite 2010) known to be infected with HIV, and 35.4% (NERCHA 2008) of those with advanced HIV infection on treatment, a critical mass of PLWHA remain under-served. In light of reductions in donor funds for ART rollout in Africa, comprehensive treatment and prevention is all the more critical.

As with any HIV/AIDS intervention, support modalities lie at the nexus of economic resources, government services, social collectivities and individual health practices. In Swaziland this nexus arises in a distinct cultural and socio-economic setting where certain practices may exacerbate the vulnerabilities many individuals, particularly women, face in their local lifeworlds. These include wife inheritance, polygamy and male sexual and reproductive entitlement to wives' younger sisters (Whiteside *et al.* 2006). They are home-based practices, moreover, that constitute the home (an extended family homestead) as an organising principle of Swazi life (Kuper 2006). For this reason, 'home' is theorised here as the physical and social space where PLWHA well-being may be most enabled or imperiled; a site that falls outside the purview of biomedically based public health research.

Shiselweni Reformed Church Home-based Care Organisation

A registered non-governmental organisation in Swaziland and South Africa, the Shiselweni Reformed Church Home-Based Care (SRC-HBC) Organisation began in 2006. The church-run project was initiated by Arnau Van Wyngaard, a theologian and South African minister with the Swaziland Reformed Church. Witnessing the impact of HIV/AIDS, he invited parishioners of his Swazi congregation to assist the many households in the community afflicted by sickness and poverty. Thirty-two individuals volunteered. Four years later, the SRC-HBC had grown exponentially to approximately 600 caregivers, serving 2500 clients in 22 communities across 100 square kilometres of Southern Swaziland. Caregivers are mostly female – though men are increasingly taking part – multi-denominational, and non-binding in religious participation.

Two seasoned caregivers have been informally trained by a volunteer nurse in HIV/AIDS education and basic first aid. They lead one-week trainings for new caregivers at the rate of about one new group every two months. The organisation is guided by scriptural maxim, 'At the Hands and Feet of Christ Serving the Community'. A South African Zulu pastor instructs modes of sharing Christian beliefs with clients. At the end of the one-week training, caregivers receive an informal certification, which culminates in a ritual whereby Mfundisi (Pastor)

Van Wyngaard bathes and washes the feet of new members to symbolise and enact the spiritual and physical caregiving roles they will serve in their communities.

The organisation is funded through small donations from individuals and religious organisations in the USA and South Africa. When available, caregivers are equipped with first aid backpacks that include a Bible. The SRC-HBC maintains vigilant data reporting processes. Caregivers record each home visitation and submit monthly reports to community coordinators. They in turn prepare reports for the regional coordinator, who details the number and gender of caregivers, the number of home visits and the number of clients, including those who are new or have moved, died, are terminal or who have chronic ailments. This information is conveyed to Pastor Van Wyngaard for oversight and to direct further health training and spiritual counselling needs.

Methods

As part of a larger medical anthropological project on religion and HIV/AIDS in Swaziland (Root 2009, 2010), started in 2005, the manuscript draws on semi-structured open-ended interviews with 20 volunteer community home-based caregivers in rural Swaziland (January and August 2009). The regional coordinator who oversaw all daily operations was also interviewed. Participants were identified through a combination of purposive and convenience sampling. The former consisted of 13 coordinators who, collectively, constituted about half of the communities served in 2009 and oversaw approximately 455 caregivers. Thus, while the number of interviews is low, the broader perspective they provided on the research question offered substantial exploratory power. Given that respondents were active in SRC-HBC groups that were diverse in the size and history of their operations, findings are felt to be reflective, though not representative, of many caregivers' experiences in the case organisation at large. Accompaniment on client home visitation, as well as extensive focused conversation with the organisation's nurse trainer and its director, provided additional primary data.

The interview schedule was operationalised to explore caregivers' motivations, perceptions of clients' needs, caregivers' HIV-related and other care practices and perceptions of the role of Christianity in home-based caregiving. English and siSwati are the official languages of Swaziland; however, residents in rural areas speak siSwati almost exclusively. Thus, because the author does not speak siSwati, when English language skills permitted, interviews were conducted one-on-one with the respondent. The remainder drew on translation assistance from fellow caregivers. Interviews were transcribed in South Africa and the USA. Given the demonstrated benefits of grounded theory analysis (Ryan and Bernard 2003, Charmaz 2006) to qualitative health research (Miller and Fredericks 1999) a grounded theory approach was used to elicit key themes from interview data. Research procedures were approved before research commenced by Baruch College's Human Research Protections Program, City University of New York (USA).

Results

Caregivers' responses to semi-structured interview questions are reported here in categories that reflect experiential patterns of providing church-run home-based care.

Motivations: love and/of knowledge

The opportunity afforded by the SRC-HBC to acquire biomedically based HIV/AIDS knowledge, and to intervene where the state fails, for example, to facilitate critical care follow-up, was a key motivator for joining the SRC-HBC. Knowledge of the organisation generally came through direct observation and word of mouth. Nocawe saw caregivers in action and asked to join, 'so I can learn about taking care of people. After they trained me, they said I can ask others interested in caregiving, so they can be trained, too'. Where some participants said they had not reached out to the afflicted prior to becoming caregivers, others recalled their struggles to extend ad hoc support to those around them. Sibusiso described how she 'would share whatever I have with sick people … Then the pastor came round to teach about [the SRC-HBC] and I saw it as an opportunity to continue helping others. Now, I feel more empowered to do so'. Cebile joined because she saw 'people suffering in different ways'. She was frustrated that she had 'no knowledge' of the diseases that plagued her community. 'That is why I volunteered myself, so that I [can] help these people and teach them what I have learned'. For Nomusa, the SRC-HBC was a chance to channel her own anguish at others' suffering: 'I volunteer, because I saw that some people [needed help] … I can't express what I feel about these people'.

Unrequited empathy emerged as a key characteristic among many participants. Asked the difference between herself and those who do not volunteer, Nomusa said it came down to deeply felt sentiments towards others' suffering: 'They don't [understand], because they don't feel what I feel about these people [who suffer]'. Specifically, the distinguishing feature was a feeling of love. 'It's because I have love', explained Futhi, 'and the love I have, I want to share with other people'.

Many participants swelled with satisfaction over their greater care competency – a competency they attributed in part to the collective problem solving that fuelled a social production of HIV care knowledge. According to Nocawe, 'Being in a group is better because you share knowledge. You may know something another person doesn't, so the care becomes better because of joint efforts and general knowledge of everybody'. Seconding the view of knowledge synergies arising from caregiver meetings, Nompumelelo explained, 'As a group it's different because every Friday we come here to report situations. We are scattered, so when we're together we share the challenges we face … We try to come with an idea how we can help'. Collective action made it possible to address a range of vulnerabilities resulting from extreme poverty. 'If I am only one person', said Nompumelelo, 'and the client needs shelter, I can't do it [alone], so we gathered together and built the client a house'. A collectivity also provided a reserve of HIV knowledge that, by knowing one another's strengths, could be drawn upon strategically. Nocawe recalled a caregiver whose client 'was on ARV [antiretroviral medications] but was given traditional medicine [too], and their abdomen became distended'. Use of traditional healing was a culture-specific challenge reported by a number of caregivers. The caregiver sought help from the group, so a second caregiver visited the client and instructed him to cease the traditional treatment and adhere to the ARV. 'Because of her knowledge', Nocawe said, 'they stopped [the traditional treatment]'.

The caregiver–client relationship

Asked how a caregiver relationship was initiated, Futhi described an ordinary introduction at the home of a potential client: 'We greet them and introduce ourselves, "We are so and so, and we are caregivers. We would like to be part of their family". We give them time to introduce themselves to us, and we start that relationship'. In different ways, caregivers also let it be known they are Christians, for example, by asking permission to pray after the introduction. Nompumelelo described how she integrated health and spiritual care practices: 'As we help clients, we also share the word of God'. Asked about clients' reactions, she said, 'Some are very excited, and others, they look as if we are just wasting our time, because we can't change them'. Whether a client identified as a Christian was no basis for withholding care; if prayer made the client uncomfortable, the caregiver would not impose it.

Interviews suggested five main reasons why a household might seek or accept caregiver services: (1) sporadic access to painkillers; (2) occasional material support; (3) assistance with household tasks, such as hauling water and preparing food; and (4) performing the most challenging of care duties, including helping clients to use the toilet and bathing them. As well, interviews suggested that caregivers were acquiring a reputation as HIV/AIDS educators who were eager to share their knowledge in non-pedantic ways. According to one participant, clients even became 'choosey', requesting one caregiver over another, apparently because the other was perceived to have more HIV knowledge. Caregiver services were readily received in Simangele's area, because the chief and his advisors, having been informed in advance by the coordinator, 'called on the people and told them about us'.

Despite the perceived benefits of home-based care, analysis suggested three reasons why households might refuse SRC-HBC outreach: First, fear that gossip had precipitated caregivers' visits. Reported Vuyisa, 'Some don't want to see a care supporter coming into their homestead without [being] invited. They ask 'Who has told you there is a sick person here? Why are you here?' Second, clients may refuse a care supporter who visited and presumably gossiped afterward. Third, caregivers sometimes belonged to the communities they served. Proximity was productive, in so far as caregiving was logistically convenient. However, the mundane tensions of neighbourly co-existence and risks of breached confidentiality could obstruct the caregiver–client relationship. Regardless, virtually every participant said that suspicion or disparagement of their care work was diminishing. Now, Futhi said, 'they can see that, really, we're doing something good'.

Caregivers' authoritative knowledge, however, was occasionally complicated by aspersions of moral superiority. According to Futhi, negativity towards caregivers could be such that 'you cannot continue with the work you are doing'. If it was felt that she had done something wrong, 'people no longer regard you as a "personal person"', a colloquialism for 'friend'. For example, if she told someone – a client or member of the community – '"If you continue doing this [e.g., drugs or alcohol], you will lose your life", they think you [think you're] better than them'. She would try to defend herself, explaining that she was not chastising the person, but rather caring for them: 'I was trying to help him to know what is good and what is not; he must decide what to do now'. Detractors accused her not only of arrogance, though, but of ignorance, pointing out that 'even if you don't drink alcohol, you still die'.

Social challenges aside, caregivers described economically impoverished conditions, which they too suffered, that often felt insuperable: 'Almost all the clients [are] dead in their life. They are too poor', reported Vuyisa. A majority of caregivers reported food shortages to be among the greatest sources of suffering and obstacles to ARV adherence. Lack of funds for clinic transport was also a pervasive problem. Clients themselves were sometimes flummoxed, unable to square caregivers' empty hands with their offers of care. Lack of material resources limited some caregivers' own self-perceived effectiveness. Nocawe lamented, 'The worst thing for me is to go to somebody without aid ... Then what do I do?' It was important to set clients' expectations. Vuyisa tried to explain to clients, 'At the moment, we don't have anything'. They mustn't expect some painkillers when they see us coming ... We don't have enough, and I don't think we'll ever have enough'. Nonetheless, her training and sense of indefatigable pathos trumped any perception that her care work was futile: 'I've saved many people. I can't stop ... Because in my family there are those with HIV...Even though there are some people that have died, I've tried my best...I spend my time, my money, my cell phone...It's impossible for me to stop now, really impossible'.

HIV/AIDS care practices

Participants estimated that much of their care work resulted from the exacerbating impact of HIV/AIDS, poverty and famine on households. Broken out here for purposes of analysis into conventional silos of HIV interventions, in reality each domain was intertwined in an ongoing caregiver–client dynamic of cultural/public health knowledge, relations and practices.

HIV testing

The first question Nomusa says she must ask a client is, 'Have you been tested?' Encouraging HIV testing, often without using the acronym itself, was a near universal practice reported by caregivers. The testing imperative was often inserted into counselling discourses of comprehensive disease testing, nesting it in more socially acceptable diagnoses. Despite her perceptions that people were better educated about HIV than in the past, Nomusa said, 'still, people won't talk about it'. Some, she added, even continued to deny HIV. So intense was fear of a positive diagnosis, explained Vuyisa, that 'even if one is sick, going to test is the last thing they do'.

Fear of HIV stigma bled into caregivers' efforts in multiple ways. Nompumelelo described how some clients asked that caregivers not use the latex gloves they are trained to use, which ran the risk of creating potentially risky situations. She explained their clinical imperative by embedding protective gloves in a caring relationship: 'We just share the idea of using gloves, that it's not that they are very sick...We try to make clear that maybe we are positive; we don't want to pass it [to them]'. By asserting that she herself might be HIV positive, Nompumelelo accomplished three enormous feats. She normalised an HIV diagnosis, preserved the client's sense of dignity and sustained the caregiving relationship.

Caregivers interacted not only with their clients but clients' families as well. Usually, Futhi said, families 'become happy because they see that you'll help them in other ways'. The participant described these 'ways', which may be highly consequential for managing the individual and household impact of HIV/AIDS, especially after ARVs are introduced. The practices are also culturally situated, reflecting the local history of the epidemic and the entrenched HIV stigma, even within families: 'We educate the family members on how to take care of the sick members'. Family members may entreat the caregiver to intervene, believing the caregiver to have a special status to the client. Futhi described a client who refused HIV testing, and whose family asked her to intervene: 'She's refusing to go', they told her. 'Maybe she will understand you…Could you please talk to her?' Futhi requested she speak with the client in private. Alone, her strategy, like other caregivers', was to normalise HIV testing by situating it within a comprehensive health seeking endeavor that often neutralised the HIV component: 'I tell them, when you're sick, you need to check everything – diabetic, or if you have TB, all those things, then include HIV testing'. Sometimes clients followed through, participants reported and sometimes not. Regardless, the caregiver in this scenario both empowered and supplemented family efforts to optimise the client's chances of survival.

ART treatment

Facilitating ART uptake and adherence were priority practices for caregivers. Like many participants, Nomusa described an integrated stepwise approach. If the client reported that they had not sought testing, but wished to do so, she offered 'by all means' to get them to a clinic. If the person had been tested, she inquired about their status. If they were HIV positive, she advised clinic follow-up. This could be a challenge: 'Some people are shy, and afraid' to seek follow-up. 'That's where you must come close to them'. If the client had commenced ART, she went to the home every day: 'What time is it? Have you taken your tablets?' If she says 'no', I say 'Remember, let's do it'.

Thulisile described a different challenge, whereby cultural and migration processes intersected in ways that could undermine clients' ART adherence: 'HIV is one of the conditions [where] ignorance is a major problem. We motivate a person to take ARVs, but after she takes the ARVs, when the festive season come, people from Joburg and all over the country [visit], they say [to the client], "No, don't take these tablets, you'd rather take this traditional medicine", and in that way we lose a lot of people, so then it's ignorance that's also a problem'. Nompumelelo echoed others who described the exacerbating combination of food insecurity and treatment, 'We encourage [clients] to follow up their treatment, but we've got people saying 'we [want to], [but] we're starving … I'm supposed to take my tablets. If I take them without food, I feel very weak'. She had helped mobilise two support groups to try to coordinate members' treatment follow-up and medication refills; a logistical hurdle to 'free' treatment that, by trying to clear it collectively, likely had secondary benefits of reducing stigma, providing psychosocial support and normalising a positive diagnosis.

Disclosure and secondary prevention

Some caregivers noticed an increasing trend towards disclosure within the caregiver–client relationship. Ascendant comfort levels appeared relative, since many participants said clients disclosed only when their family was not present. 'It's not easy for them to tell us', Nomusa said, 'but the way we are talking with them, now they are telling us ... That's why we try to give them some gloves ... or soap'. Talking was itself a salient care practice. Caregivers wove empathic compassion with concrete counsel. Said Sibusiso, 'If somebody confides in me [who is HIV positive], I keep it discreet, and we discuss and hug each other. I don't even tell my family. I don't even tell my children. It's between me and my client'. Managing HIV disclosure was among the most complex roles that caregivers assumed. 'Talking' was a primary means of eliciting and conveying vital HIV information, especially following a disclosure: 'Some of them are very brave. They say, "Eh, my friend, I've went for checking [testing], and unfortunately, I'm HIV positive. Now where do I go?"' Vuyisa advises going to the voluntary counselling and testing (VCT) centres and preparing to start ARVs. 'But if you don't want to start on ARVs you must listen to what [clinic personnel tell] you to do, and be very careful ... Keep on checking the CD4 count'.

Tholakele described how she handled fears of abandonment and disparagement clients sometimes felt they risked, if they disclosed to family members: '[The client] tells you their secret, so...you give her that love'. Because she cannot be with the client around the clock, she advises the client to 'tell one of your family members who is going to be with you almost seven days a week'. If a client asks Tholakele to assume that task of telling them, she declines and instructs the person to name a family member. Tholakele calls for that person: 'I say, "This one is very sick, as you know, but now they know their status ... So he just needs help from you at times"'. Many caregivers counselled the importance of disclosing to sexual partners, as well. 'It's important that the partner must know', Futhi told her clients, 'so that they have protected sex and help each other [e.g., remind you to take your drugs]'. Sibusiso described a softer approach, counselling that they 'must try and tell their sexual partners – it's difficult, but at times, eventually you find that some [have] opened up to each other'.

Gender vulnerabilities and home-based care

Some husbands' resistance to HIV testing, and obstructions to wives' attempts at HIV care were challenges many caregivers faced. The nurse trainer explained: 'It becomes very difficult for us. I've got a typical case. He hasn't tested, but it's typical that [he] may be positive, but when we ask him to test, he says the [wife] must go and test. If ever she is found positive, she will have to pack her bags and go'. Futhi described an HIV positive woman whose husband was aware of his wife's status and that she was on ARVs, whereas he was not. One day, when the woman was away from home, she returned to find that her husband had thrown her medications down the toilet. 'The woman became very sick', recalled Futhi. 'She waited for a long period [to return to] clinic for more tablets; they were busy fighting and talking'. Asked about recurring reports of men's apparently greater reluctance to test, Nocawe said, 'Men are just like that; they prefer to die rather than go on ARV'. Her own son, she said, had been put on ART, yet he refused to take them: 'He says he'd rather die than take so many tablets'. In some instances, though, vulnerabilities were successfully resolved with home-based brokering strategies not possible in a clinic setting. Futhi had a female client who had commenced ART, but the husband, despite knowing his wife's status, refused testing. Futhi told her, 'We'll find a day to visit when [you and your husband] are together, and [I'll] educate about HIV and AIDS, how to use safe sex – all those things'. Afterward, the caregiver returned to find that the husband had finally agreed to test.

Religion and home-based care

An important aim of the interview design was to understand caregivers' views on the signifiance of being a Christian in providing home-based care. 'This work needs somebody who knows about Jesus', Nomusa explained. Pressed, she concretised what it meant 'to know' Jesus in her world: 'It's because you have to be faithful. If you give me something to give my clients [e.g., food], I must do that. If I'm not faithful, I will eat it myself. If I tell my clients, "I will come to you at nine o'clock", [and I'm not there], the client will [doubt me]'. The rhetoric of religion became a discourse of love, and then a care practice, since the care work itself could be off-putting. 'You can't be a caregiver when you don't have love', she insisted. 'You can't, because some clients are so sick they can't go to the toilet, so you have to help them'. This could include cleaning up diarrhoea and using her own money to wash clients' linens. In short, being faithful to a Christian ethos of Jesus' love was enacted and experienced as a seemingly boundless faithfulness to clients' needs. Identifiable by the group's mustard coloured jersey, inscribed with the group's scriptural maxim, caregivers like Nomusa felt households were more receptive than in the past: 'They call me even if I am away. People need me'. At the same time, it was an activity that chagrined some community members. Some called her a 'fool' for working for nothing. Asked how a spirit of volunteerism could grow in such an environment, Nompumelelo felt that teaching gospel could help to create 'that spirit of pity in someone', a precursor to the compassion that appeared to enable all caregivers' practices.

Although HIV/AIDS knowledge was acquired through training, 'love' and 'talk' were paramount care practices that benefited by modelling. With prior HIV/AIDS training from a Lutheran Development Center, the SRC-HBC asked Vuyisa to 'accompany [caregivers] to clients' homes to show them how to speak to [sick] people'. Cultivating 'love' and 'talk' among caregivers was also necessary to create a cohesive care group, which was essential for extending care to clients. Asked about the challenges of coordinating 49 caregivers, Nomusa intimated that caregivers are still people amongst whom tensions can arise. One of her biggest challenges was to get caregivers to 'love one another', a task she undertook by having them 'talk, talk, talk'. She explained, 'Everything – we have to start with the Bible'. Such love was 'something [they said they] didn't have before'. But since becoming volunteer caregivers, they told her, 'We are getting love, loving other people thinking about helping someone'.

Caregiving and care of self

Given the little research that exists on caregivers' well-being, the schedule included questions about participants' health and who takes care of them. The question often elicited a chuckle at the irony that caregivers might be uncared for. However, a number of participants said that their SRC-HBC peers did. One of the strengths of a semi-structured format is the dialogic space it creates for respondents to reconfigure the interview question itself. This occurred when Sibusiso explained how she looks after her own well-being. She began by saying she uses the protective gloves; she then segued to the subjects of marriage and abstinence: 'As it is, I wasn't likely to be married, but now I just abstain from everything and stay with my children'. Christianity served as a resource for self-preservation of body and spirit: 'My faith is keeping me going, because I believe I'm the temple of God. I've got to keep myself clean and safe. That's how I keep myself going'. Asked whether she felt abstinence could really prevent HIV in Swaziland, she wove Christian teachings with public health imperatives: 'It's going to be very difficult for people, but I preach this. Each time we meet, I try to preach to the caregivers that we need to abstain, because this [body] is the temple of God ... But we also need to abstain because of the diseases that are around. Some are beginning to follow the example, but some still find it very difficult to stay without men'. She then proceeded to indict marriage on public health grounds, detailing its risks to women. 'What's the use of going around sleeping with a man, when you know the marriage is not going to last? It's very shaky ground ... Like, you're in a marriage that can break tomorrow. What's the purpose?' She was frustrated that she could think of no strategy that a married woman could deploy to refuse sex, since bride price rendered her his family's property. 'But those who are not married?' she concluded, 'It's not worthwhile'.

Discussion

Theoretical framework

By situating clinical phenomena in locale-specific constellations of social experience (Bolton and Singer 1992) that are often marked by structural vulnerabilities (Farmer 2001), medical anthropology is uniquely well suited to generating new insights on HIV/AIDS and religion at multiple levels (Pfeiffer 2005, Dilger 2007). The concept of RHA helps to deepen this inquiry with the notions of tangible assets, understood as 'compassionate care, material support and health provision', and intangible assets, described as 'spiritual encouragement, knowledge giving and moral formation' (ARHAP 2006, p. 3). In some regards, RHA can be understood as social capital. However, because RHA also encompasses religious identities, social networks and ideologies (Olivier *et al.* 2006), findings from this study demonstrated how RHA offers considerably greater explanatory power than social capital concepts alone. These findings suggest compelling public health relationships, analysed below, between diverse aspects of religion and caregivers' perceived impact on individual, household and community well-being – impacts *in situ* to the local research area, and also, possibly, to vulnerable settings with similar structural, cultural and epidemiological profiles.

HIV/AIDS knowledge: training and empowerment

To theorise religion and public health dynamics in sub-Saharan Africa (SSA), RHA, as an emergent concept, benefits by research that documents the diverse kinds of AIDS work that religious entities undertake in different settings (Schmid *et al.* 2008, p. 3). Such documentation was a key aim of this study. As a religious organisation originating in one local congregation, the SRC-HBC provided much-desired opportunities for HIV/AIDS training. The HIV/AIDS-related care practices caregivers described, and their religious consciousness of these practices, suggested activities with substantial public health significance. Their reports of the most critical HIV-related decision-making processes an individual faces (testing, disclosure, treatment uptake, gender vulnerabilities and pressures to use traditional healing) constituted empirical data of both client needs and the tangible 'compassionate care' and intangible 'knowledge giving' assets that the SRC-HBC mobilised as a response. And unlike sporadic non-contextual HIV/AIDS slogans and well-scripted clinic counselling, participants' reports of HIV education in familiar church settings, in groups assembled under trees, and one-on-one indicated 'the impact that religio-cultural frameworks' (ARHAP 2006, p. 5) may have by transforming HIV information into real-time actionable knowledge – a response to community (and individual) suffering that often felt meaningful and effective.

An expanding literature has profiled community caregivers serving as ARV and TB treatment supporters in SSA (Weidle *et al.* 2006, Apondi *et al.* 2007). Studies of community home-based care (CHBC) (Ncama and Uys 2006, Shaibu 2006, Ncama 2007) and HIV/AIDS care continuums (Uys 2003, Thomas *et al.* 2006) have suggested that, properly designed and supported, different forms of home-based care may address a range of PLWHA needs. Ideally, home-based and community-based care would help to provide palliative relief from the physical pain of HIV-related cancers and, unlike formal health care services, tend to the daily psychosocial and spiritual challenges patients and their families face (Sepulveda *et al.* 2003). Despite the urgency of local needs and potential wealth of assets inherent in CHBC (Olenja 1999), little is known of the operational challenges these diversely constituted groups face (Mohammad and Gikonyo 2005). According to participants in this study, treatment support required caregivers have basic knowledge of ART, acknowledge the limits of their knowledge and work within material and social constraints. Showing up the limits of silo-constructed HIV interventions, caregivers often described clients' disclosures as intensely private moments that precipitated highly consequential decisions for household relations and HIV health practices.

Single service home-based care is distinguished by its volunteer operations (Van Dyk (2005) summarised in Mulenga 2007, pp. 111–112) and church-run modalities in particular by members' shared scriptural ethos of empathic engagement with others' suffering (Mulenga 2007). This engagement, involving people, relationships and emotions reflects the proposition by Olivier *et al.* (2006) that 'what often makes RHAs different from other health associations, institutions or structures lies in what is not visible – the volitional, motivational and mobilising capacities that are rooted in vital affective and symbolic dimensions of religious faith, belief and behaviour' (p. 11). Thus, compared with VCT counselling, this study's caregivers, having already established special relationships, were strategically positioned to explain and re-explain pre- and post-diagnosis practices at a pace, and in a place, that heeded clients' HIV understanding, emotions and personal circumstances. Moreover, cognisant of clients' potential vulnerabilities, especially those faced by wives, some caregivers endeavored to broker safer disclosure between sex partners. To address these public health challenges, caregivers innovated a purposive, culturally situated strategy of 'talk' and 'coming close'; a step-wise approach to enculturating a spectrum of HIV health practices. Such practices constituted uniquely situated HIV interventions beyond the geographic reach of formal health care. They were public health practices, moreover, whose framing context was discursively articulated in Christian terms, of serving communities and alleviating suffering.

Leveraging assets: religion and social transformations in care/knowledge

Opportunities for HIV/AIDS training alone did not explain SRC-HBC's rapid expansion. Religious identity, leadership and scriptural ethos emerged as part and parcel of HIV/AIDS care and demonstrated the synergies of tangible and intangible RHA. Interpreted by the director, the Bible's paramount lesson was the love of giving freely (voluntarily and unconditionally) – a subjective emotion and care practice that cross-cut many interviews. Its maxim communicated a grounding ideology and guiding ethos that integrated volunteerism and HIV care. From a public health perspective, the heuristic distinction between ideology and ethos is important, first, to situate the group's evangelical aspects in a local setting, and second, to begin to identify potential collaborative challenges between religious and non-religious health entities. As an ideology, defined as a 'body of doctrine [...]' along with the devices for putting it into operation',[2] evangelism was a discursive feature of SRC-HBC training in so far as, explained the director, it '[helps caregivers] to speak about their faith in such a way that people can understand the message, yet do not feel they are being forced into "repenting" – as so often happens'. As an ethos, the maxim reflected the 'character or disposition of a community, group, [or] person'.[3] In this study, the collective disposition was to 'love' freely and unconditionally.

From participants' perspectives, this religious ethos was an indispensable feature of caregiving – a finding that augments the core meaning of asset in RHA, understood as an 'endogenous' resource that can be 'leveraged and grown' in the service of public health (Haddad et al. 2008, p. 4). Subjective and agentive experiences, such as those described in this study, are critical data that bear on enacting endogenous assets. Faced with overwhelming suffering and chronic shortages of food and medicine, caregivers struggled with their care limitations. They were supposed to be 'caring', yet they often had nothing to give. A deeply felt Christianity helped assuage this troubling disconnect. Lacking food or painkillers for clients, Nocawe said, 'Really, you can't cope [as a caregiver], unless you've got a heart to do it'. Asked how religion provided that 'heart', she explained that in faith or religion, you pray to get the strength to go on, 'and even if you don't have anything, when you get to the patient you can pray; that's a pillar of strength for me'.

Caregiver reports suggested that the SRC-HBC was transformative for many individuals and the communities they served. The feedback loop of knowledge acquisition and action through caregiving had become a discursive feature of a caregiver identity. 'How can I stop home-based care?' one participant said. 'I think, what must I do now? I need more training'. By identifying the substantive functionality that 'love' and 'talk' played as culturally situated care practices, this study surfaced deeply felt experiences of self that, in turn, suggested new notions of personhood. This reflexivity, moreover, conveyed ways that religious consciousness and HIV training were leveraged as care 'interventions' and intimated a self and social transformation that likely would not have developed in the absence of a scriptural ethos and church-run organisational structure. Communities directly witnessed SRC-HBC caregivers in action, igniting discussion of hidden agendas, moral superiority and admiration; all elements in an alchemy of sociocultural change. 'When I'm dressed like this [the group's jersey]', said Sibusiso, 'people start being attracted to me, and I tell them who I am and what [I do]'. Asked what people actually see, she detailed care tasks that were simultaneously mundane and sacred: 'They see how we help other people. If you're not able to fetch water, we go to the river for you. If you're unable to wash yourself, we wash you. People look at us ... "We would like to be like them"'. Witnessing caregivers' work, Sibusiso said, was having the effect of converting some individuals 'because of what we're doing'.

It is important to grasp that these public care practices are enacted in a society marked by considerable HIV stigma (Dlamini *et al.* 2007, Root 2010). At the same time, they transpire in domestic spaces conceptualised in the sociological literature as private. They are practices, moreover, discursively articulated in Christian terms. Witnessing caregivers' work, she said, was having the effect of converting some individuals 'because of what we're doing'. To the extent that this may be the case across the organisation's 22 communities, the SRC-HBC response to collective suffering may transform aspects of religion, and religion, in turn, transform aspects of HIV/AIDS. This transformation was conceptualised by many in this study as a religious ethos of selfless love, made real through practices that offered ongoing support to clients and caregivers alike. The shift – from individuals extending ad hoc care to teams of caregivers who were attributed with important health skills – seemed to give rise to a new subjectivity: a state of mind of 'how to be' under conditions of extreme suffering; a caregiving self-astute to the diversity and complexity of client relationships; a sensitivity to others' needs and their own limitations; and supportive peer relationships that did not exist before.

Religiosity as a feature of RHA is little explored. Asked how long she would be a caregiver, Nomusa answered, 'Until I die, because when I die being a caregiver, I will die in Christ'. Christianity provided the foundation for Sibusiso's pro-sexual abstinence stance as a form of self-care; however, it did so in ways that would likely be unrecognisable to most scholars. Sibusiso leveraged its empowering aspects in sociocultural environments where church is often one of the only sites where women congregate on a regular basis outside the home (Taylor 2006), and in doing so problematised reductive notions of Christianity as exclusively oppressive of women. In the USA, in particular, sexual abstinence often is the Maginot Line that defines whether a researcher or policy-maker is a progressive or conservative voice in AIDS programming. Yet, despite investigation into other social aspects of HIV/AIDS, the multiple meanings that sexual abstinence might have in distinctive cultural settings have engaged little research. That Sibusiso counselled sexual abstinence, using a mélange of religious and biomedical discourses, to members of a church-run HBC group is potentially culturally transformative. It featured a woman in a poor rural area publicly denouncing the institution of marriage in Swaziland, because of the risks of infection she said it poses. Sexual abstinence for her was positioned as a protest against male sexual prerogatives. This is a distinctly different abstinence discourse than in the USA. Hers was a rationale in religious and culture-specific terms that most AIDS researchers, by virtue of the latter's 'local' culture-specific politics, have neglected to investigate.

Conclusion

This manuscript contributes to an expanding body of peer-reviewed research that examines the multifactorial significance of religion to subjective experiences of and community responses to HIV/AIDS, especially local churches, whose institutional presence far exceeds those of formal health care settings in many areas of the world. On a programmatic level, a deeper understanding of how religious entities engage HIV/AIDS, operationally and ideologically, is necessary to strengthen multisectoral collaboration (Olivier *et al.* 2006, p. 59). Designed to collect experiential data from caregivers who volunteer with a church-run home-based care organisation, the study generated insights on the tangible and intangible assets that were mobilised to assist hard-hit communities in Swaziland and the subjective experiences of doing so. The organisation's RHA 'portfolio' included a dynamic constellation of leadership, organisation, networks, practices and identities. Where generosity and caregiving certainly were not unknown prior to the SRC-HBC, the formalisation of these characteristics, the scale at which they are practiced and their public enactment traced the outlines of new categories of personhood that challenge the HIV/AIDS status quo of sickness and stigma.

Overall, the interviews provided a compelling picture of essential site-specific conversations around HIV/AIDS that happen on clients' own terms, in their own spaces, in order to navigate the material constraints and gender vulnerabilities that many faced. Analysis of how caregivers engaged these challenges shed light on the limitations of an inadequate health system whose clinical milieus cannot eliminate entirely the fear, reluctance and distrust that often mediate daily health practices. Finally, the significance to caregivers of acquiring and enacting HIV/AIDS knowledge as part of a scriptural ethos *of* pathos foreground some of the shortcomings of authoritative public health discourses around religion and HIV/AIDS. In addition to furthering research on RHA, such data are essential to nuance debates that have arguably impeded deeper investigation of Christian religion and HIV/AIDS in Africa. Studies are needed to further document and theorise the ways in which conservative religious discourses in one cultural setting, resituated in another, may become progressive in innovative ways that could strengthen HIV/AIDS programming.

Notes

1. Participants' quotes have been edited for clarity and word count. Efforts were made to retain as much of intended meanings as possible.
2. Dictionary.com. *Dictionary.com Unabridged*. Random House, Inc. Available from: http://dictionary.reference.com/browse/ideology [Accessed 19 June 2011].
3. Dictionary.com. *Dictionary.com Unabridged*. Random House, Inc. Available from: http://dictionary.reference.com/browse/ethos [Accessed 19 June 2011].

References

Adogame, A., 2007. HIV/AIDS support and African Pentecostalism: the case of the Redeemed Christian Church of God (RCCG). *Journal of Health Psychology*, 12, 475–484.

African Religious Health Assets Programme (ARHAP), 2006. *Appreciating assets: the contribution of religion to universal access in Africa. Mapping, understanding, translating and engaging religious health assets in Zambia and Lesotho in support of universal access to HIV/AIDS treatment, care and prevention.* Cape Town: ARHAP.

Agadjanian, V. and Sen, S., 2007. Promises and challenges of faith-based AIDS care and support in Mozambique. *American Journal of Public Health*, 97, 362–366.

Allen, T. and Heald, S., 2004. HIV/AIDS policy in Africa: what has worked in Uganda and what has failed in Botswana? *Journal of International Development*, 16 (8), 1141–1154.

Apondi, R., Bunnell, R., Awor, A., Wamai, N., Bikaako-Kajura, W., Solberg, P., Stall, R., Coutinho, A. and Mermin, J., 2007. Home-based antiretroviral care is associated with positive social outcomes in a prospective cohort in Uganda. *Journal of Acquired Immune Deficiency Syndrome*, 44 (1), 71–76.

Becker, F. and Geissler, P.W., 2007. Searching for pathways in a landscape of death: religion and AIDS in East Africa. *Journal of Religion in Africa*, 37, 1–15.

Bolton, R. and Singer, M., eds., 1992. *Rethinking AIDS prevention: cultural approaches.* Philadelphia, PA: Gordon and Breach Science.

Central Statistical Office (CSO) [Swaziland], and Macro International Inc., 2008. *Swaziland demographic and health survey 2006–2007.* Mbabane, Swaziland: Central Statistical Office and Macro International

Charmaz, K., 2006. *Constructing grounded theory: a practical guide through qualitative analysis.* Los Angeles, CA: Sage.

Cochrane, J., 2006. Religion, public health and a church for the 21st century. *International Review of Mission*, 95 (376/377), 59–72.

Dilger, H., 2007. Healing the wounds of modernity: salvation, community and care in a neo-Pentecostal church in Dar es Salaam, Tanzania. *Journal of Religion in Africa*, 37, 59–88.

Dlamini, P., Kohi, T., Uys, L., Phetihu, R., Chirwa, M., Naidoo, J., Holzemer, W., Greef, M., and Makoae, L., 2007. Verbal and physical abuse and neglect as manifestations of HIV/AIDS stigma in five African countries. *Public Health Nursing*, 24, 389–399.

Farmer, P., 2001. *Infections and inequalities: the modern plague.* Los Angeles, CA: University of California Press.

Gifford, P., 2008. Trajectories in African christianity. *International Journal for the Study of the Christian Church*, 8 (4), 275–289.

Haddad, B., Olivier, J., and De Gruchy, S., 2008. *The potential and perils of partnership: Christian religious entities and collaborative stakeholders responding to HIV and AIDS in Kenya, Malawi and the DRC.* Study commissioned by Tearfund and UNAIDS. Interim report. ARHAP. Available from: http://www.arhap.uct.ac.za/publications.php [Accessed 20 May 2011].

HIV InSite, 2010. *Swaziland comprehensive indicator report.* San Francisco, University of California. Available from: http://www.hivinsite.ucsf.edu/global?page=cr09-wz-00& post=19&cid=WZ [Accessed 2 May 2010].

Joint United Nations Programme on HIV/AIDS (UNAIDS). November, 2009. *2009 AIDS epidemic update.* Geneva: Joint United Nations Programme on HIV/AIDS (UNAIDS) and World Health Organization (WHO).

Kuper, H., 2006. *The Swazi: a South African kingdom.* New York: Holt, Rinehart and Winston.

Meyer, B., 2004. Christianity in Africa: from African Independent to Pentecostal-Charismatic churches. *Annual Review of Anthropology*, 33 (1), 447–474.

Miller, S.I. and Fredericks, M., 1999. How does grounded theory explain? *Qualitative Health Research*, 9 (4), 538–551.

Mohammad, N. and Gikonyo, J., 2005. *Operational challenges: community home-based care for PLWHA in multi-country HIV/AIDS programs for Sub-Saharan Africa.* Africa Region Working Paper Series, No. 88. The World Bank Group.

Mulenga, K.C., 2007. *Empowering church-based communities for home-based care: a pastoral response to HIV/AIDS in Zambia.* Thesis (Masters). Faculty of Theology. University of Pretoria. [Now in book form: Publisher, VDM Verlag 2009].

National Emergency Response Council on HIV/AIDS (NERCHA), 2008. *Monitoring the declaration of commitment on HIV/AIDS (UNGASS). Swaziland country report.* Mbabane, Swaziland: The Government of the Kingdom of Swaziland, January 2008. Available from: http://www.data.unaids.org/pub/Report/2008/swaziland_2008_country_progress_report_en. pdf [Accessed 6 May 2010].

National Emergency Response Council on HIV/AIDS (NERCHA), 2010. *Monitoring the declaration of the commitment on HIV and AIDS (UNGASS). Swaziland country report.* UNAIDS, March 2010.

Ncama, B.P., 2007. Acceptance and disclosure of HIV status through an integrated community/home-based care program in South Africa. *International Nursing Review,* 54, 391–397.

Ncama, B. and Uys, L., 2006. Community impact of HIV status disclosure through an integrated community home-based care programme. *African Journal of AIDS Research,* 5 (3), 265–271.

Olenja, J., 1999. Assessing community attitude towards home-based care for people with AIDS (PWAS) in Kenya. *Journal of Community Health,* 24 (3), 187–199.

Olivier, J., Cochrane, J., and Schmid, B., 2006. *ARHAP literature review: working in a bounded field of unknowing.* Cape Town: African Religious Health Assets Programme.

Pan African Christian AIDS Network (PACANet), 2008. *Situational analysis: Swaziland report.* Available at: http://pacanetusa.com/search?keywords=swaziland [Accessed 19 May 2011].

Pfeiffer, J., 2005. Commodity fetishismo: the Holy Spirit, and the turn to Pentecostal and African Independent Churches in Central Mozambique. *Culture Medicine and Psychiatry,* 29 (3), 255–283.

Root, R., 2009. Being positive in church: religious participation and HIV disclosure rationale among people living with HIV/AIDS in rural Swaziland. *African Journal of AIDS Research,* 8 (3), 295–309.

Root, R., 2010. Situating PLWHA experiences of HIV-related stigma in Swaziland. *Global Public Health,* 5 (5), 523–538.

Ryan, G.W. and Bernard, R.H., 2003. Techniques to identify themes. *Field Methods,* 15, 85–109.

Schmid, B., Thomas, E., Olivier, J., and Cochrane, JR., 2008. *The contribution of religious entities to health in sub-Saharan Africa.* Study funded by Bill & Melinda Gates Foundation. Unpublished report. ARHAP. Available from: http://www.arhap.uct.ac.za/publications.php [Accessed 20 May 2011]

Sepulveda, C., Habiyambere, V., Amandua, J., Borok, M., Kikule, E., Mudanga, B., Ngoma, T., and Solomon, B., 2003. Quality care at the end of life in Africa. *British Medical Journal,* 327 (408), 209–213.

Shaibu, S., 2006. Community home-based care in a rural village: challenges and strategies. *Journal of Transcultural Nursing,* 17 (89), 89–94.

Taylor, N., 2006. *Working together? Challenges and opportunities for international development agencies and the church in the response to AIDS in Africa.* Tearfund HIV and AIDS Briefing Paper No. 7. Middlesex, UK: Tearfund.

Thomas, L., Schmid, B., Gwele, M., Ngubo, R., and Cochrane, J., 2006. *'Let us embrace': the role and significance of an integrated faith-based initiative for HIV and AIDS.* ARHAP research report: Masangane case study [Eastern Cape, South Africa]. Cape Town, South Africa: African Religious Health Assets Programme.

UNAIDS, WHO, UNICEF, 2008. *Epidemiological fact sheet on HIV and AIDS: core data on epidemiology and response – Swaziland. 2008 update.* Geneva: The UNAIDS/WHO Working Group on Global HIV/AIDS and STI Surveillance.

Uys, L.R., 2003. Aspects of the care of people with HIV/AIDS in South Africa. *Public Health Nursing,* 20, 271–280.

Van Dyk, A., 2005. *HIV/AIDS & counselling: a multidisciplinary approach.* 3rd ed. Cape Town, South Africa: Maskew Miller Longman.

Weidle, P.J., Wamai, N., Solberg, P., Liechty, C., Sendagala, S., Were, W., Mermin, J., Buchacs, K., Behumbiize, P., Ransom, R., and Bunnell, R., 2006. Adherence to antiretroviral therapy in a home-based AIDS care programme in rural Uganda. *Lancet*, 368, 1587–1594.

Whiteside, A., Andrade, C., Arrehag, L., Dlamini, S., Ginindza, T., and Parikh, A., 2006. *The socio-economic impact of HIV/AIDS in Swaziland*. Mbabane, Swaziland: National Emergency Response Council on HIV/AIDS (NERCHA) and Health Economics and HIV/AIDS Research Division.

World Bank Group, 2010. *Swaziland. World development indicators database*. December 2010. The World Bank Group. Available from: http://web.worldbank.org/WBSITE/EXTERNAL /COUNTRIES/AFRICAEXT/SWAZILANDEXTN/0,menuPK:375134 ~ pagePK:141132 ~ piPK:141109 ~ theSitePK:375023,00.html [Accessed 21 May 2011].

Conflicts between conservative Christian institutions and secular groups in sub-Saharan Africa: Ideological discourses on sexualities, reproduction and HIV/AIDS

Joanne E. Mantell[a], Jacqueline Correale[a], Jessica Adams-Skinner[a] and Zena A. Stein[a,b]

[a]HIV Center for Clinical and Behavioral Studies, New York State Psychiatric Institute and Columbia University, New York, NY, USA; [b]GH Sergievsky Center, Mailman School of Public Health, Columbia University, New York, NY, USA

Religious and secular institutions advocate strategies that represent all points on the continuum to reduce the spread of HIV/AIDS. Drawing on an extensive literature review of studies conducted in sub-Saharan Africa, we focus on those secular institutions that support all effective methods of reducing HIV/AIDS transmission and those conservative religious institutions that support a limited set of prevention methods. We conclude by identifying topics for dialogue between these viewpoints that should facilitate cooperation by expanding the generally acceptable HIV/AIDS prevention methods, especially the use of condoms.

Introduction

Societies have traditionally granted broad authority to religious institutions to create and oversee rules for many aspects of individual behaviour, including those affecting sexuality, the role of women, reproduction, health education and care of the sick. Yet, religious institutions vary in how they view these issues. Some rely on Holy Books for their authority and are resistant to change, while others are morally closer to liberal secular groups. Because HIV/AIDS risk-reduction is inextricably intertwined with the rights to sexual and reproductive autonomy as well as freedom from discrimination of sexual orientation and gender, societal policies and actions on HIV prevention are divisive. In this article, we focus on sub-Saharan African conservative churches and their leaders who support only those HIV/AIDS prevention methods proscribed by Holy Writ (Pfeiffer 2004) and tradition. We compared this prevention approach to the approach of groups we characterise as secular and who accept all HIV/AIDS prevention methods as a human right. Conservative religious organisations include Evangelical, Fundamentalist, Charismatic, Pentecostal and Roman Catholic churches.

In the last two decades, conservative Christian institutions, sometimes spurred by government funding, have imposed their moral judgements on HIV/AIDS prevention (Gusman 2009, Prince *et al.* 2009). Conservative religious and secular institutions have disagreements concerning abstinence, premarital and extramarital sex, contraception and homosexuality. The resulting clashes are identified in our literature review of published English-language and grey literature between 1995 and 2011. We searched electronic databases, including PubMed, Medline/PsychInfo, ProQuest, American Theological Library Association, Humanities, New/Old Testament abstracts, Religious & Theological abstracts and Google; terms included: religious institutions; reproduction and sex; religious institutions and condoms; religious institutions, conception and HIV; as well as human rights and religion. We also reviewed the bibliographies of all articles to identify additional references. This process yielded a total of 100 articles. We conclude this analysis with a discussion of how secular and conservative religious institutions might join together to increase HIV/AIDS prevention initiatives.

Secular and religious collisions regarding sexual and reproductive rights

Early Hebrews linked reproduction with survival (Yarber 2010), disapproving of all sexual activity not aimed at reproduction. Many conservative Christian institutions maintain adherence to this restrictive perspective (Marsden 2006, Bottum 2008). Secular institutions, drawing upon philosophy, moral reasoning and science (Center for Health & Social Policy 2005), believe that the four sexual human rights – sexual autonomy, access to HIV/AIDS risk-reduction information, reproductive autonomy, as well as freedom from stigma and discrimination of sexual orientation and gender – are needed for effective HIV prevention. Some conservative Christian institutions have adopted limited revisions of their traditional approaches to sexual and reproductive health behaviours in response to the HIV/AIDS epidemic. As Gordon and Mwale (2006, pp. 71–72) state: 'Faith-based organisations have always struggled with how to marry their moral mission and the need to protect health and life, given the reality of people's sexual lives'. The teachings of religious institutions on moral issues are in theory universal and unchanging. Professor of Philosophy Lamont (2010, p. 24) at the University of Notre Dame in Australia states, 'there is no sociological theory or sociological evidence to support the claim that religions can preserve or increase their influence while lowering their standards and submitting to the society around them'. He observes that mainstream Protestant churches that make few demands on their members are declining, whereas more demanding Evangelical and Pentecostal churches are growing in sub-Saharan Africa. In practice, this concern with the consequences of 'lowering' standards has led conservative religious institutions to resist any change for fear of diminishing the size of their congregations.

Unsurprisingly, neither conservative Christian institutions nor secular groups accept the other's definition of sexual and reproductive rights. As Bayes and Tohidi (2001, p. 5) note: 'The struggle is between those who define gender roles and sexuality on a fixed hierarchical order, often sanctioned by religious doctrinal necessity, as predetermined by divine and/or natural order, and those who view these as matters of social-historical construction and individual choice'. We believe that it is important to help the conservative religious teachers to limit the spread of HIV/ AIDS.

Linking sexual and reproductive health with a 'human rights' perspective has broadened the secular discourse from being judgemental (AIDS is punishment for sexual immorality) to embracing empowerment and challenge of social injustices (Schmid 2006). The landmark 1994 International Conference on Population and Development (ICPD) and 1995 Beijing Platform of Action at the Fourth World Conference on Women signified for many a global secular recognition of sexual and reproductive health rights. These rights have been reaffirmed by many other groups, such as the World Health Organization, United Nations Population Fund and the Protocol on the Rights of Women in Africa (Center for Reproductive Rights 2006). A landmark decision by the Human Rights Committee in Australia in 1994, Toonen v. Australia, argued that non-discrimination provisions regarding sex included sexual orientation (Saiz 2004). In 2007, the Yogyakarta Principles on the Application of Human Rights Law in relation to Sexual Orientation argued for the protection of privacy rights for all, regardless of sexual orientation or gender identity (O'Flaherty and Fisher 2008).

Although secular organisations hold that reproductive and sexual rights (e.g., abortions for HIV-positive pregnant women) should be universal, some conservative religious institutions actively contest these 'human rights' (Miller 2000). The manner in which countries tackle these issues is dependent on laws enacted to address local secular and religious values. For some of these secular groups, the refusal of Catholicism and Islam to condone family planning and abortion is based on their shared vision of women as inferior and men as in charge (Kissling 1994–1995), and perhaps also on social control of sexuality.

Below, we explore how religious doctrines of conservative churches frequently conflict with the four 'human rights'. We present biblical citations that these churches rely upon and findings from empirical studies.

The right to sexual autonomy

Heterosexual sex within marriage is the accepted, if not celebrated, expression of sexuality within the vast majority of Christian traditions (Louw 2008). A number of passages in the New Testament speak to the sanctity of marriage and prohibitions against sex outside of marriage.

> Marriage [is] honourable in all, and the bed undefiled: but whoremongers and adulterers God will judge. (Hebrews 13:4, King James Version, http://kingjbible.com/hebrews/13. htm)

> Now the works of the flesh are manifest, which are these, adultery, fornication, uncleanness, lasciviousness....they which do such things shall not inherit the kingdom of God. (Galatians 5:19-21, King James Version, http://kingjbible.com/galatians/5.htm)

According to conservative churches, the only HIV/AIDS prevention method condoned by these biblical passages is sexual activity within marriage (Obaid 2005, Morgan 2009). Pre-marital abstinence and marital fidelity, the only acceptable norms, vary greatly with culture, tradition and economy (Benn 2002).

Unfortunately, with the demands of separation for work, exemplified by migrant labour and military service, the preservation of fidelity has seldom proved realistic and considerable research on sexually transmitted infections bears evidence to this (Lurie *et al.* 2003). Multiple Demographic and Health Surveys in sub-Saharan Africa indicate that sex with a non-spouse or non-cohabiting partner is common – e.g., 11% among Nigerian men (Mitsunaga *et al.* 2005), 19% among married Zambian men (Kimuna and Djamba 2005) and 21% among Cameroonian (Kongnyuy and Wiysonge 2007) and South African men (South African Department of Health 2007).

Interpretations regarding sexual autonomy vary by and within Christian denominations. In Evangelical, African Independent and Mainline churches, many of which are fervent in their adherence to traditional interpretations of the New Testament, extramarital sex is viewed as a sin that imperils salvation (Gennrich 2004). In Smith's study (2004, p. 430) of rural–urban migrant Igbo Nigerian youth, Pentecostal and other 'Born Again' pastors viewed HIV/AIDS as a 'scourge visited by God on a society that has turned its back on religion and morality'. In the words of one of Smith's female participants,

> . . . this place is like Sodom and Gomorrah. Nigerians are being punished for their sins. If people did not have sex here and there, if the society were not so corrupt, there would be no AIDS. . . Yes, it is God's punishment, but we have brought it on ourselves.

Smith (2004) categorised the religious views affecting sexual behaviour among these Nigerian youth as abstinence, moral partnering (sexually active but based on monogamy and religion) and denial (pre- and extra-marital relationships are rationalised, hidden and denied). Unfortunately, the youth who adopted moral partnering were convinced that they were unconcerned about HIV/AIDS (because they trusted their partners also to limit their relationships) and therefore did not need to use condoms with a moral partner.

Some conservative Christian churches frame sexual intercourse as a sacred aspect of life, viewing it as a manifestation of God who evokes his presence within the sexual union of each married couple. Pre-marital sex is a defined sin; pre-marital virginity is equated with purity. Pre-marital sex, homosexual sex and sex work are labelled by many conservative Christian churches as failures of the flesh, sins of impurity. Members of these religious communities who choose to adopt any of these behaviours unsurprisingly do not seek information on protecting themselves from HIV for fear of exclusion from their church (Denis 2009).

The willingness of Christian pastors to incorporate HIV/AIDS messages into their sermons varies widely. In 85 churches and mosques in rural Malawi, about 30% of religious services referred to HIV/AIDS (Trinitapoli 2006). Abstinence and fidelity were the second most common themes to those of repentance and salvation. Indigenous Church leaders in an urban area in KwaZulu-Natal, South Africa, recognised the need to speak about HIV/AIDS, but were reluctant to discuss this topic from the pulpit because of cultural constraints in talking about sex in a public forum. Similarly, in an ethnographic study of university students from an urban Pentecostal Church in Kampala, Uganda, the ideals of abstinence and fidelity were preached (Sadgrove 2007). In the words of one pastor:

Sin is a big problem to God and Christians. The condomised culture is becoming normal but we stick to abc — Abstinence, Be faithful, Christ! — as the answer. People pump it 'it's ok as long as you use condoms'. No! the condom culture is not the kingdom culture.

Religious condemnation of sex outside marriage is believed to be effective in reducing sexually transmitted HIV infection (Gregson *et al.* 1999, Garner 2000). Through in-depth interviews and household visits, Garner (2000) examined the effects of conservative Christian institutions on members' sexual behaviour in a peri-urban community in KwaZulu-Natal, South Africa. He outlined four mechanisms used by these religious institutions: (1) indoctrination; (2) fostering moral conformity through participation in church activities and mobilising social capital through youth groups and camps; (3) maintaining fidelity through fear of exclusion; and (4) educating its followers. The importance of the four mechanisms varied across denominations and time. Pentecostal church members had significantly lower levels of extra- and pre-marital sex and were the least likely to have an illegitimate child. Similarly, in a study in Malawi, male members of Pentecostal churches had a lower level of perceived HIV risk and risk behaviours (Trinitapoli and Regnerus 2006). In Ghana (Luginaah *et al.* 2005) and in East Africa (Gusman 2009, Parsitau 2009), mandatory HIV testing has been used by some churches for couples intending to marry so as to 'save innocent men and women'. However, Campbell *et al.* (2010) noted that such social control can be a double-edged sword, reinforcing and maintaining gender relations that disadvantage women's ability to negotiate safer sex. This contradiction was also noted in Sadgrove's (2007) study of Pentecostal university students in Kampala, Uganda, as well as Mate's (2002) study of Pentecostal churches in Zimbabwe.

One key unanswered question is whether strict norms about pre-marital abstinence and marital fidelity and advocacy for the ideal of sexual restraint result in less risky behaviour among members of conservative religious institutions. The studies described above suggest that membership in Evangelical/Pentecostal churches may be protective against HIV; however, the pathways to explain the links between HIV risk perceptions and risk behaviour are unknown. There are several possible reasons to support this protective effect, including negative consequences of nonadherence to behavioural expectations of no sex outside of marriage; indoctrination into church's world view of strict moral codes and socialisation within restricted social networks; and social control.

The right to HIV/AIDS risk-reduction information

The consensus at the 2001 United Nations General Assembly Special Session on AIDS was that there is the need for a comprehensive package of HIV/AIDS risk-reduction interventions. This call was ignored by the Bush administration in excluding all scientific references to the efficacy of condoms from US government programmes and websites (Meckler 2002, Human Rights Watch 2004). This omission served to increase scepticism among public, religious and governmental institutions about which components of the ABC approach (Abstain, Be Faithful, and Condom Use) to HIV/AIDS prevention should be endorsed (Green *et al.* 2006).

There appear to be two reasons why conservative Christian religious institutions continue to oppose condom use. The first is that many rely on statements in the Old

Testament, e.g., be fruitful and multiply (Tharao *et al.* 2006), while secularists believe that the biblical proscription to flourish is better achieved by restricting the quantity and quality of childbearing. Since condoms remain a key component of all HIV prevention strategies endorsed by secular groups, we analyse the objections to their use in relation to contraception; to promiscuity; to sex education in the young; to church leadership; and to harm-reduction for HIV. Lastly, we consider signs of variation and change in the positions of some religious groups.

Religious opposition to condoms

Clement of Alexandria (AD195) wrote, 'Because of its divine institution for the propagation of man, the seed is not to be vainly ejaculated, nor is it to be damaged, nor is it to be wasted' The Catholic Church refined this concept 60 years ago when it promulgated 'natural' family planning ('rhythm method') as the only approved means of regulating procreation (Pope Pius XII 1951). However, introduction of the effective birth control pill 50 years ago revolutionised family planning, as many perceived it to be more protective and sexually satisfying than the rhythm method.

The second reason they oppose condom use is the fear it will encourage promiscuity (Krakauer and Newbery 2007, Foster *et al.* 2009, Aguwa 2010). In a world with lifetime mutual monogamy, virtually all sexually transmitted diseases would be eliminated. Unfortunately, throughout recorded human history, societies have been unsuccessful in imposing this stance.

Condoms and sex education for the young

Conservative Christian religious institutions that promote abstinence and fidelity believe that these practices prevent new infections, frequently citing Uganda as the exemplary model (Denis 2003). Programmes, whether school-based or government-sponsored, that promote abstinence-only are out of touch with the reality that many young people throughout sub-Saharan Africa are sexually active before marriage, and these programs withhold access to comprehensive sex education (Santelli *et al.* 2006). For example, nearly 40% of women and 40–45% of men in sub-Saharan Africa have had sex by age 18, and more than 75% of women and more than 60% of men, by age 20 (Biddlecom *et al.* 2007). Clear evidence is found in many societies that abstinence-only programmes are less effective in delaying or reducing teenage pregnancy than are 'abstinence plus' programmes that use a hierarchical approach that promotes abstinence first but also condoms and contraceptive information (Perrin and DeJoy 2003, Dworkin and Santelli 2007, Kirby *et al.* 2007). This is good news for preventing teenage pregnancy as well as for reducing disease transmission. The inflexibility of religious precepts of conservative Christian churches suggests the need for secular groups, e.g., schools, to encourage educators to refine their definitions of moral precepts to protect young people against AIDS. Restrictions on access to HIV/AIDS information and condoms impede public health and, in turn, the right to protect health (Human Rights Watch 2004).

A Seventh Day Adventist Church in Zimbabwe punished five youth members by suspending them from a gathering when condoms were discovered in their cabins. This church believes that condom use leads to promiscuity, which is seen as a violation of the sixth commandment (Makahamadze and Sibanda 2008). As the Pastor and camp's Youth Director said, 'If the health workers come to teach about HIV and AIDS and the risks associated with it, I will welcome them. But if they talk about condoms, I will tell them to go to hell'.

Church leadership

Interviews conducted with 117 church ministers, lay leaders, people living with HIV/ AIDS (PLWHA) and caregivers of PLWHA from 30 Mainline, Pentecostal/ Evangelical and African Independent churches in Pietermaritzburg, South Africa, showed that ministers and lay leaders were far less accepting of condom use than PLWHA or their caregivers (Gennrich 2004). Two-thirds of ministers and half of lay leaders opposed condom distribution in church halls. In addition, ministers and lay leaders did not consider condoms to be a useful strategy for preventing HIV/AIDS, although a few did suggest that congregants use condoms. Among PLWHA, 11 viewed their churches as promoting condoms, 9 believed their churches opposed condom promotion and 13 said their churches were silent about their position on condom use. Discussions with PLWHA and their caregivers indicated that even though they were more accepting of condom use, distribution of condoms would conflict with the churches' message of abstinence and recipients might be labelled as promiscuous. In 16 semi-structured interviews on HIV prevention with Catholic, Evangelical Lutheran and the Assemblies of God clergy in South Africa, religious leaders faced three dilemmas in their approach to HIV/AIDS prevention messages: the clergy's breaking the silence on HIV/AIDS; HIV/AIDS prevention messages being misconstrued by or inappropriate for young people; and gender different-prevention messages (Eriksson *et al.* 2010). These interviews indicated that talking openly about sex, HIV and condoms – 'unbiblical things' – might provoke conflict between the church leaders and the church hierarchy and resistance from congregants. To break this silence, some church leaders reported they encouraged HIV testing during pre-marital counselling, but expressed ambivalence about HIV prevention messages for youth due to the belief that parents are responsible for such sexual education and the taboo of talking about sex in public venues. Church leaders with negative attitudes about condoms would support condom use only among married HIV-discordant couples and people who were non-church goers. Leaders with positive attitudes cited 'taking precaution' and 'using protection' rather than mention the word 'condom'. Although church leaders claimed that they believed in gender equality, the HIV prevention messages some promoted were contradictory, e.g., that only a woman needs to be 'strong enough' to refuse sex with men other than their spouse.

Variation and change in religious institutions

In his first visit to Africa in 2009, Pope Benedict XVI stated that HIV/AIDS cannot be overcome through the distribution of condoms. More recently, the Pope's stance on denouncing condom use in all cases as an instrument of immorality has shifted to accepting the need for condoms for reducing the risk of infection in some circumstances, such as by male sex workers (Donadio and Goodstein 2010, Holden 2010). The Pope's current position is a demonstration that the Catholic Church can change its moral reasoning in response to people's health issues. Yet, even with the

Pope's acceptance, some church leaders, such as the Cardinal of the Kenyan Catholic Church, continue to vociferously oppose condom use for any reason (PlusNews 2011). Others in Africa have taken a 'don't ask, don't tell' approach to condom use, where the church is seen as 'promoting prostitution' if it allows people to use condoms. And even though most churches do support condom use, it is with the understanding that each individual must choose for themselves. Similarly, Father Chris Townsend of the South African Catholic Bishop's Conference said, 'In South Africa it's our approach that we will teach people about condoms. We don't encourage them but we don't discourage them'. Father Townsend's rationale, which was supported by a number of African Catholic priests, that not opposing is not encouraging condom use, observes the form of the doctrine of Papal condemnation of general condom use (Kardas-Nelson 2009). Governmental HIV prevention strategies may conflict with religious organisations, as illustrated in a study of mainstream Christian, Pentecostal and Muslim religious leaders in Malawi (Rankin *et al.* 2008). Interviews with 40 religious leaders from five institutions indicated that the government's promotion and distribution of condoms as part of the ABC approach were in direct opposition to the stance of all religious institutions on pre-marital abstinence and marital fidelity, characterised as the 'condom divide'. Their condemnation of condoms was based on the belief that promoting condom use gives people the license to sin and threatens the moral values central to their faith. Similarly, the Jeito brand condom social marketing campaign became a source of contention with religious leaders in Mozambique who viewed condom promotion as clashing with hegemonous church morality (Pfeiffer 2004).

Harm-reduction

Some leaders of conservative Protestant churches in rural Malawi equate condom use with being 'Satanic' (Trinitapoli 2006, 2009). Other religious leaders were more accepting of condom use as a contraceptive for marital partners and for people unable to abstain from sex, though they seldom preached this message from the pulpit. In Kenya, some Islamic religious leaders, relying on the 'lesser of two evils' principle, permit the use of condoms based on their benefit of reducing the spread of AIDS (Maulana *et al.* 2009). Commitment to a harm-reduction concept has also been reported in a study of church leaders and congregants in Pietermaritzburg, South Africa (Gennrich 2004). As one congregant reported,

> We are losing people we love and care for. We know condoms are not 100% safe but we are committed to reducing the spread of the virus. [Our] Canon... helped me to sort out my thinking about condoms. He is very clear that condoms are important for all – including married couples – and they are not just a license for promiscuity, but a sensible tool to reduce the risk of spreading HIV in a society that puts all kinds of pressures on people to engage in sex, whether it is their choice or not.

In light of the high number of HIV infections within Southern Africa, the South African Catholic Bishop's Conference asked the Vatican to review the stance on condoms as a preventive measure, 'particularly in situations where one person in a marriage is HIV-positive, and the other is HIV-negative', says Father Townsend (Kardas-Nelson 2009).

The right to reproductive autonomy

Religion plays an essential role in how people understand and make choices about contraception, fertility, motherhood and abortion. Many Christians interpret the New Testament as valuing the dignity of every person, love and compassion of God and the rights and responsibilities of members of a society. The Catholic Church encourages reproduction within marriage, but is not explicit, and is even self-contradictory, in its position towards non-reproductive sex. For example, is sex permissible for the sole purpose of pleasure? The Bible encourages sexual pleasure:

> Let her be as the loving hind and pleasant roe; let her breasts satisfy thee at all times; and be thou ravished always with her love. (Proverbs 5:19, King James Version, http:// kingjbible.com/proverbs/5.htm)

> ...Let him kiss me with the kisses of his mouth: for your love is better than wine. (Song of Solomon 1:2, King James Version, http://kingjbible.com/songs /1.htm)

Catholic ideology maintains that sex is only allowed for procreation purposes, but peculiarly approves the rhythm method. Other than abstinence, Catholics are likely to have difficulty reconciling Humanae Vitae Encyclical and the advice by secularists given to HIV-positive individuals about sexual decisions. How do HIV-discordant couples prevent the spread of HIV/AIDS to their uninfected partner and their unborn foetus? Married HIV-positive individuals unaware of their partner's HIV status, and women who unintentionally become pregnant face the complexity of dealing with the HIV status of a foetus.

Mate's ethnographic study (2002) of Pentecostalism in two women's organisations in Zimbabwe describes how the 'Born Again' discourse exalts motherhood, viewing it as God's work, God's plan for women, God making miracles and surrendering to God. In contrast, contraceptive use is defined as breaking the shroud of motherhood. Thus, Pentecostal religious ideology considers all pregnancies to be desirable and abortion a non-viable option. This deification of fertility denies women control over their bodies. Fertility is viewed as a way to sustain marriage and demonstrate self-worth, whereas infertility and miscarriage are associated with being the devil's work and a justification for men to divorce, have multiple marriages and engage in extramarital sex.

Secular groups deem it appropriate for both partners to have equal rights to decide family size. Decisions are reached in the context of our understanding of biology and, to a lesser extent, demography and social sciences. From a 'human rights' perspective, women's ability to control their fertility could reduce maternal and child mortality (Freedman et al. 2005).

The right to freedom from stigma and discrimination of sexual orientation and gender

Sexual orientation

Conservative religious institutions often promulgate rigid norms of sexual identity (Horn 2010), supported by an ideological stance that homosexuality is sinful. The Old Testament clearly condemns homosexuality.

Thou shalt not lie with mankind, as with womankind: it is abomination. (Leviticus 18:22, King James Version, http://kingjbible.com/leviticus/18.htm)

Religious traditions are often used to justify laws and judicial decisions as well as discrimination against sexual minorities (EHAHRDP 2007). Policies and laws have been adopted that exclude protection of the individual rights of people based on their sexual orientation (Twiss 1998). According to the International Lesbian and Gay Association, among 242 countries, 78 have laws that criminalise male same-sex relationships and in 45, female same-sex relationships are illegal (International Lesbian, Gay, Bisexual, Trans and Intersex Association 2008). In parts of sub-Saharan Africa, authorities relying on religious laws impose whipping, life imprisonment and even death penalties. When same-sex relationships between consenting adults are criminalised, fear of jail, violent attacks, stigma and discrimination reduce the number of gay people who choose to be tested for HIV.

Although alternative sexualities are known to have existed in sub-Saharan Africa for at least 400 years, many people today have highly negative attitudes towards sexual minorities, attributed to both retained colonial laws and values and powerful religious beliefs (Oxfam 2010). Two widely publicised events provoked a secular outcry in support of same-sex partnerships in sub-Saharan Africa (Senior 2010). The first occurred in Malawi, a deeply conservative society where traditional religions are mixed with the values of the Anglican Church. Based on the country's 'decency' law, a 14-year jail sentence for sodomy was imposed on two homosexual men who underwent a same-sex commitment ceremony, but they subsequently received a presidential pardon. There are proposals to penalise those who engage in homosexual behaviour in Zimbabwe's new Constitution (Radio Vop Zimbabwe 2010), a country which has historically used state power to restrict sexual rights and citizenship and denigrate homosexuality (Phillips 2004). Religiously encouraged laws such as these continue to create conflict between conservative religious institutions and secular groups. The second and more egregious situation relates to the proposed Bahati anti-homosexuality bill in Uganda first introduced in October 2009, discussed, but rejected in Parliament in May 2011. However, it could potentially be carried over into the next session of Parliament (Kron 2011, International Gay & Lesbian Human Rights Commission 2011a), which seeks to establish comprehensive legislation (ostensibly) to protect the traditional family by prohibiting any form of same-sex relations, allegedly spurred by the actions of US Evangelicals. This anti-homosexuality bill calls for imprisonment for those engaging in same-sex relations as well as for those members of the public who fail to report such activities, with the original draft calling for the possibility of life imprisonment and the death penalty by serial offenders or HIV-positive individuals (Civil Society Coalition on Human Rights and Constitutional Law 2009, Harris *et al.* 2010, NY Daily News 2010, International Gay & Lesbian Human Rights Commission 2011b). In a terribly sad turn of events, Mr. David Kato, a Ugandan gay-rights activist was beaten to death in his home on 26 January 2011, three weeks after he won a court case against a local newspaper that published the names and addresses of gay-rights campaigners in the East African nation (Bloomberg News 2011).

There is a tug of war in sub-Saharan Africa between those countries attempting to impose penalties on homosexuals and those countries, such as South Africa,

Namibia and Botswana, eager to improve societal health by recognising the rights of homosexuals, especially as it relates to the fight against HIV/AIDS. Conservative Christian churches rely on literal interpretation of the Bible to deal with sin, which may allow them to separate themselves from the 'pollution' of the world. Liberal Christian churches focus on brotherly love and compassion. Christians pride themselves on doing things that Jesus Christ would do if He were here now, and many believe that Christ would condemn injury, let alone murder, based on sexual orientation. When church leaders in Tanzania were asked how they confront HIV/AIDS and its stigma, one pastor said, 'If God is going to judge us on how we treated people with AIDS, we didn't do very well. May God forgive us' (Hartwig *et al.* 2006).

Gender

Religious institutions have historically been involved in the roles of men and women in society. Many conservative churches place women in dependent, submissive roles, justified by selected interpretation of biblical texts (Marshall and Taylor 2006). This conservative gender ideology impedes the control of HIV/AIDS when pervasive male hierarchical control is reflected in women having secondary status in society. HIV prevention messages that promote fidelity for a woman, regardless of a man's unfaithfulness, may effectively be a death sentence for women whose partners refuse to use condoms. Evangelical churches rely on a literal interpretation of 'wives, submit yourselves unto your own husbands, as it is fit in the Lord' to identify 'appropriate' gender-role expectations. For example, Agadjanian (2005), Agadjanian and Menjívar (2008) found differences in these standards and expectations for men and women in many churches in Mozambique. Condom use was likely to be discussed at men's meetings, but was unlikely to be discussed at women's meetings. Women congregants (especially those from healing churches) reported they were reminded that having an extramarital relationship could result in the loss of property rights and children. Women congregants had many traditional responsibilities, e.g., care for the sick, but were rarely allowed to assume pastoral leadership positions in African Evangelical churches.

Crumbley (2003) studied the attitudes towards women from three different churches in Nigeria. The Christ Apostolic Church prohibits women from being ordained. In the Celestial Church of Christ, women are not only prohibited from being ordained, but from entering the altar area or the church during menstruation. Although women in the Church of the Lord are prohibited from entering the church while menstruating and their participation in discussions of theological matters is limited since they are viewed as being ritually impure, they can be ordained but cannot perform Holy Communion, weddings or baptism before they are menopausal or reach the age of 60.

In Malawi, responsibility for translating religious doctrine into practice is placed in the hands of men, effectively serving to control and subordinate women's work and sexuality. Not only do Malawian women receive fewer benefits than men from religious institutions, but they lack support from them (Rankin *et al.* 2005, p. 11). 'If the man strays from the marriage, we say the wife should forgive him; if the woman strays, then the man should divorce her'. As with discrimination against sexual orientation, so the diminution of women at many levels in conservative religious institutions, although less recognised, is a serious obstacle to HIV prevention. Women are, in fact, too often seen as the vectors rather than the victims of HIV.

Opportunities and challenges to collaboration

Fostering problem-solving through critical consciousness (Freire 1970) and enhanced dialogue would help secular groups and Christian religious institutions join in implementing the four 'human rights' we have postulated as relevant to HIV prevention. It is as difficult for conservative religious institutions to consider changing their view of sexual and reproductive rights as it is for secular organisations to accept religious theology and doctrine. Neither religious absolutism nor secular free spirit will lead them to work harmoniously in reducing HIV/AIDS. Although the differences between conservative Christian institutions and the secular groups are too complex to be resolved in the short-term, we encourage both groups to begin by being clear where they are on the continuum between respect for religious doctrines and 'human rights'. Interestingly, a Center for Health & Social Policy Report for the John D. and Catherine T. MacArthur Foundation and the Ford Foundation (Center for Health & Social Policy 2005) noted that only one secular organisation was working exclusively at the intersection of religion and sexual/reproductive health in Africa.

As to sexual autonomy, reproductive autonomy and tolerance of deviance, we recommend adopting Wingood's (2010) diplomatic approaches to congregants of religious organisations through organised church groups. This could take the form of meetings of small groups of women or families, guided by individuals who are neither religious nor secular leaders. These discussions should be constructive in helping to frame responses to these universal transgressions against the current conservative Christian ideals of sexual autonomy, reproductive autonomy and tolerance of deviance.

While in religious terms sex outside of marriage is 'sinful', in the secular world it is often condemned as a personal betrayal with potential loss of property rights. In fact, the punishment, even when only social disgrace, may be more hurtful in secular groups than the price of forgiveness in religious groups. When considering sexual autonomy, both secularists and religious groups must remind themselves of the injunction of Jesus, '. . . he that is without sin among you, let him first cast a stone at her' (John 8, King James Version, http://kingjbible.com/john/8.htm).

Secularists must devote themselves to convincing conservative religious institutions that many will not and cannot change their practices in reproductive autonomy. Individuals who have opted to have children outside marriage or fewer children in marriage could respectfully explain their decision to selected groups of congregants.

Stigma and discrimination are the most immutable of the four issues. Intolerance to social deviance of any kind is universal among secularists and religious congregants. Secularists must convince those conservative Christian religious institutions which consider homosexuality as socially or biologically deviant that acceptance or forgiveness is an appropriate Christian ideal. What is urgently needed is a dialogue that emphasises the convergence of religious institutions and secular groups to promote social justice, avowed by all.

Smith (2009) argues that even in the case of unfaithfulness to one's spouse/ partner, God's righteousness and mercy make the use of condoms to prevent HIV a Christian ethical responsibility. Drawing upon the Protestant theology, Smith argues that religion and condoms for disease prevention are linked because of the Christian obligation to protect life. Revision by the Catholic Church of its ideological stance from no condom use to condoning condom use for disease prevention in limited circumstances is encouraging. As Winfield (2010) writes about Pope Benedict's stance on condoms, 'condom use in some cases could be a first step toward a more moral and responsible human sexuality ... to diminish the risk of contagion'.

As promotion of condom use is the most effective method of reducing the spread of HIV, we propose that these parties concentrate on what seems achievable in the short-term:

(1) Selecting local people, e.g., tribal chiefs and political leaders who are experienced, to help plan and implement HIV prevention programmes and testing events.
(2) Encouraging people living or working with HIV/AIDS to serve as brokers between conservative religious institutions, liberal Christian institutions and secular organisations. By personalising HIV/AIDS, they can help all to become more accepting of condom use.
(3) Inspiring conservative religious leaders to provide HIV prevention messages, emphasising from the pulpit that God's righteousness and mercy, Christ's mission of forgiving, warrant appropriate condom use. It is an ethical responsibility for church leaders to teach that if church members cannot control their 'sinful' sexual activity, using condoms would dramatically reduce HIV risk.
(4) Mobilising liberal churches to discuss with conservative religious congregants their common religious responsibility to compel broader condom use. Teaming up liberal and conservative churches may be more acceptable than secular groups teamed with conservative churches because of trust and credibility within the commonality of religious organisations.
(5) Encouraging liberal Christian religious institutions and secular groups to join in discussions of condom use with conservative religious institutions in every available forum.
(6) Emboldening secular leaders to enhance their understanding of how the Bible relates to condom use, perhaps participating in bible studies at conservative Christian churches.
(7) Encouraging conservative Christian churches to hold discussions in which public health practitioners illustrate that condom use will reduce the number of sexually transmitted diseases as well as offspring from 'sinful' sexual relations.

In the longer-term, all of the above strategies should be employed to help integrate theology with 'human rights' relating to sexual autonomy, HIV/AIDS risk-reduction information, reproductive autonomy, as well as freedom from stigma and discrimination of sexual orientation and gender. Biomedical technologies that do not limit pregnancy – antiretrovirals and medical male circumcision for HIV prevention – may become more acceptable than condoms. Given steps like the Pope's tweaking of Christian theology as to condom use, we are optimistic that people of good will join together to reduce the spread of HIV.

Acknowledgements

This study was supported by a centre grant from the National Institute of Mental Health to the HIV Center for Clinical and Behavioral Studies at the New York State Psychiatric Institute and Columbia University [P30-MH43520; Principal Investigator: Anke A. Ehrhardt, PhD] and the *Eunice Kennedy Shriver* National Institute of Child Health and Human Development [R01-HD054303; Principal Investigator: John J. Chin, PhD]. The views and opinions expressed in this article are solely those of the authors and do not necessarily represent the official view of the National Institute of Mental Health and the *Eunice Kennedy Shriver* National Institute of Child Health and Human Development.

References

Agadjanian, V., 2005. Gender, religious involvement, and HIV/AIDS prevention in Mozambique. *Social Science & Medicine*, 61, 1529–1539.

Agadjanian, V. and Menjívar, C., 2008. Talking about the 'epidemic of the millennium': religion, informal communication, and HIV/AIDS in sub-Saharan Africa. *Social Problems*, 55, 301–321.

Aguwa, J., 2010. Religion and HIV/AIDS prevention in Nigeria. *Crosscurrents*, 60, 208–223.

Bayes, J.H. and Tohidi, N., 2001. *Globalization, gender, and religion*. New York: Palgrave.

Benn, C., 2002. The influence of cultural and religious frameworks on the future course of the HIV/AIDS pandemic. *Journal of Theology for Southern Africa*, 113, 3–18.

Biddlecom, A.E., Hessburg, L., Singh, S., Bankole, A., and Darabi, L., 2007. *Protecting the next generation in sub-Saharan Africa: learning from adolescents to prevent HIV and unintended pregnancy*. New York: Guttmacher Institute.

Bloomberg News. 2011. Ugandan-gay-rights-activist-is-killed-by-unknown-attackers. Available from: http://www.bloomberg.com/news/2011-01-27/ugandan-gay-rights-activist-is-killed-by-unknown-attackers.html [Accessed 27 Jan 2011].

Bottum, J., 2008. The death of Protestant America: a political theory of the Protestant mainline. *First Things: A Monthly Journal of Religion & Public Life*, August/September. Available from: http://www.firstthings.com/article/2008/08/001-the-death-of-protestant-america-a-political-theory-of-the-protestant-mainline-19 [Accessed 11 May 2011].

Campbell, C., Skovdal, M., and Gibbs, A., 2010. Creating social spaces to tackle AIDS-related stigma: reviewing the role of church groups in sub-Saharan Africa. *AIDS & Behavior*, doi: 10.1007/s10461-010-9766-0.

Center for Health & Social Policy. 2005. *Religion and sexual and reproductive health and rights: an inventory of organizations, scholars, and foundations*. A report to The John D. and Catherine T. MacArthur Foundation and The Ford Foundation. Available from: http://www.chsp.org/Religion_and_Sexual_and_Reproductive_Health_and_Rights.pdf [Accessed 31 Aug 2010].

Center for Reproductive Rights. 2006. The protocol on the rights of women in Africa: an instrument for advancing reproductive and sexual rights. Available from: http://www.reproductiverights.org [Accessed 13 Aug 2010].

Civil Society Coalition on Human Rights and Constitutional Law, December 2009. Uganda's anti-homosexuality bill. The great divide. Available from: http://www.ugandans4rights.org/downloads/09_12_18_Anti-homosexuality_Bill_Compilation.pdf [Accessed 8 May 2011].

Crumbley, D.H., 2003. Patriarchies, prophets, and procreation: sources of gender practices in three African churches. *Africa*, 73 (4), 584–605.

Denis, P., 2003. Sexuality and AIDS in South Africa. *Journal of Theology for Southern Africa*, 115, 63–77.

Denis, P., 2009. The church's impact on HIV prevention and mitigation in South Africa: reflections of a historian. *Journal of Theology for Southern Africa*, 134, 66–81.

Donadio, R. and Goodstein, L., 2010. In rare cases, Pope justifies use of condoms. *New York Times*, 20 November. Available from: http://www.nytimes.com/2010/11/21/world/europe/21pope.html [Accessed 13 Dec 2010].

Dworkin, S. and Santelli, J., 2007. Do abstinence-plus interventions reduce sexual risk behavior among youth? *PLoS Medicine*, 4, 1437–1439, e276. doi:10.1371/journal.pmed.0040276

EHAHRDP (East and Horn of Africa Human Rights Defenders Project). 2007. Defending human rights: a resource book for human rights defenders. Available from: http://www.defenddefenders.org/documents/Defending Human Rights A Resource Book.pdf [Accessed 6 Jan 2011].

Eriksson, E., Lindmark, G., Axemo, P., Haddad, B., and Maina Ahlberg, B.M., 2010. Ambivalence, silence and gender differences in church leaders' HIV-prevention messages to young people in KwaZulu-Natal, South Africa. Culture. *Health & Sexuality*, 12, 103–114.

Foster, G., Mwase-Kasanda, C., Maswere, E., and Winberg, C., 2009. A purpose-driven response: building united action on HIV/AIDS for the church in Mozambique. *African religious health assets (ARHAP) conference*, 13–16 July, Cape Town, South Africa.

Freedman, L.P., Waldman, R.J., de Pinho, H., Wirth, M.E., Mushtaque, A., Chowdhury, R., and Rosenfield, A., 2005. Transforming health systems to improve the lives of women and children. *Lancet*, 365, 997–1000.

Freire, P., 1970. *Pedagogy of the oppressed*. New York: Continuum.

Garner, R.C., 2000. Safe sects? Dynamic religion and AIDS in South Africa. *The Journal of Modern African Studies*, 38, 41–69.

Gennrich, D., 2004. *Churches and HIV/AIDS: exploring how local churches are integrating HIV/AIDS in the life and ministries of the church and how those most directly affected experience these. Research report*. Pietermaritzburg: Project Pietermaritzburg Agency for Christian Social Awareness (PACSA). Available from: http://www.pacsa.org.za [Accessed 21 Aug 2010].

Gordon, G. and Mwale, V., 2006. Preventing HIV with young people: a case study from Zambia. *Reproductive Health Matters*, 14, 68–79.

Green, E.C., Halperin, D.T., Nantulya, V., and Hogle, J.A., 2006. Uganda's HIV prevention success: the role of sexual behaviour change and the national response. *AIDS and Behavior*, 10, 335–346.

Gregson, S., Zhuwau, T., Anderson, R.M., and Chandiwana, S.K., 1999. Apostles and Zionists: the influence of religion on demographic change in rural Zimbabwe. *Population Studies*, 53, 179–193.

Gusman, A., 2009. HIV/AIDS, Pentecostal churches, and the 'Joseph generation' in Uganda. *Africa Today*, 57, 67–86.

Harris, D., Hinman, K., and Karamehmedovic, A., 2010. Anti-homosexual bill in Uganda causes global uproar. ABC NEWS/Nightline. Available from: http://abcnews.go.com/Nightline/anti-homosexuality-bill-uganda-global-uproar/story?id = 10045436 [Accessed 25 Jun 2010].

Hartwig, K.A., Kissioki, S., and Hartwig, C.D., 2006. Church leaders confront HIV/AIDS and stigma: a case study from Tanzania. *Journal of Community & Applied Social Psychology*, 16, 492–497.

Holden, A., 2010. Analysis: what the Pope really said about condoms. Catholic News Agency. Available from: http://www.catholicnewsagency.com/news/analysis-what-the-pope-really-said-about-condoms/ [Accessed 13 Dec 2010].

Horn, J., 2010. Christian fundamentalisms and women's rights in the African context: mapping the Terrain. Available from: http://www.awid.org/eng/About-AWID/AWID-Initiatives/Resisting-and-Challenging-Religious-Fundamentalisms/CF-Case_Studies [Accessed 19 Jan 2011].

Human Rights Watch, 2004. *Access to condoms and HIV/AIDS information: a global health and human rights concern.* New York, NY: Human Rights Watch. Available from: http://www.hrw.org/en/reports/2004/11/30/access-condoms-and-hivaids-information [Accessed 2 Jan 2011].

International Lesbian, Gay, Bisexual, Trans and Intersex Association, 2008. *Material on state sponsored homophobia in world.* Available from: http://ilga.org/ilga/en/article/1195 [Accessed 2 Oct 2010].

International Gay & Lesbian Human Rights Commission, 2011a. IGLHRC shocked at possible passage of Ugandan anti-homosexuality bill. Available from: http://www.iglhrc.org/cgi-bin/iowa/article/pressroom/pressrelease/1384.html [Accessed 15 May 2011].

International Gay & Lesbian Human Rights Commission, 2011b. *Uganda update: IGLHRC welcomes closing of Ugandan parliament without vote on anti-homosexuality bill.* Available from: http://www.iglhrc.org/cgi-bin/iowa/article/pressroom/pressrelease/1390.html [Accessed 31 May 2011].

Kardas-Nelson, M., 2009. *Catholics, condoms and confusion.* Available from: http://www.mg.co.za/article/2009-03-27-catholics-condoms-and confusion [Accessed 29 July 2010]

Kimuna, S.R. and Djamba, Y.K., 2005. Wealth and extramarital sex among men in Zambia. *International Family Planning Perspectives*, 31, 83–89.

Kirby, D.B., Laris, B.A., and Rolleri, L.A., 2007. Sex and HIV education programs: their impact on sexual behaviors of young people throughout the world. *Journal of Adolescent Health*, 40, 206–217.

Kissling, F., 1994. 1995. The challenge of Christianity. *American University Law Review*, 44, 1345–1349.

Kongnyuy, E.J. and Wiysonge, C.S., 2007. Alcohol use and extramarital sex among men in Cameroon. *BMC International Health and Human Rights*, 7, 6. doi:10.1186/1472-698X-7-6

Krakauer, M. and Newbery, J., 2007. Churches' responses to HIV/AIDS in two South African communities. *Journal of International Association of Physicians in AIDS Care*, 6, 27–35.

Kron, J., 2011. Antigay bill in Uganda is shelved in Parliament. *The New York Times*, A17.

Lamont, J., 2010. The prophet motive. *First Things*, 219, 21–24.

Louw, D.J., 2008. Beyond 'gayism'? Towards a theology of sensual, erotic embodiment within an eschatological approach to human sexuality. *Journal of Theology for Southern Africa*, 132, 108–124.

Luginaah, I.N., Yiridoe, E.K., and Taabazuing, M.M., 2005. From mandatory to voluntary testing: balancing human rights, religious and cultural values, and HIV/AIDS prevention in Ghana. *Social Science & Medicine*, 61, 1689–1700.

Lurie, M.N., Williams, B.G., Zuma, K., Mkaya-Mwamburi, D., Garnett, G.P., Sturm, A.W., Sweat, M.D., Gittelsohn, J., and Abdool Karim, S.S., 2003. The impact of migration on HIV-1 transmission in South Africa: a study of migrant and nonmigrant men and their partners. *Sexually Transmitted Diseases*, 30, 149–156.

Makahamadze, T. and Sibanda, F., 2008. 'Battle for survival': responses of the seventh-day adventist church to the HIV and AIDS pandemic in Zimbabwe. *Swedish Missiological Themes*, 96, 293–310.

Marsden, G.M., 2006. *Fundamentalism and American culture.* 2nd ed. New York: Oxford University Press.

Marshall, M. and Taylor, N., 2006. Tackling HIV and AIDS with faith-based communities: learning from attitudes on gender relations and sexual rights within local evangelical churches in Burkina Faso, Zimbabwe, and South Africa. *Gender & Development*, 14, 363–374.

Mate, R., 2002. Wombs as god's laboratories: pentecostal discourses of femininity in Zimbabwe. *Africa*, 72, 549–568.

Maulana, A.O., Krumeich, A., and Van Den Borne, B., 2009. Emerging discourse: Islamic teaching in HIV prevention in Kenya. Culture. *Health & Sexuality*, 11, 559–569.

Meckler, L., 2002. HIV prevention groups say Bush administration is targeting their work. Available from: http://www.actupny.org/reports/cdc-condoms.html [Accessed 3 Oct 2010].

Miller, A.M., 2000. Sexual but not reproductive: exploring the junction and disjunction of sexual and reproductive rights. *Health and Human Rights*, 4, 68–109.

Mitsunaga, T.M., Powell, A.M., Heard, N.J., and Larsen, U.M., 2005. Extramarital sex among Nigerian men: polygyny and other risk factors. *Journal of Acquired Immune Deficiency Syndromes*, 39, 478–488.

Morgan, R., 2009. Religion and HIV/AIDS policy in faith-based organizations. *African Religious Health Assets Programme (ARHAP) conference*, 13–16 July, Cape Town, South Africa. Leeds, United Kingdom: University of Leeds, 1–15.

NY Daily News. 2010. Ugandan anti-homosexuality bill won't be dropped: parliament speaker. Available from: http://www.nydailynews.com/news/world/2010/03/02/2010-03-02_ugandan_antihomosexuality_bill_wont_be_dropped_parliament_speaker.html [Accessed 25 Jun 2010].

Obaid, T.A., 2005. Religion and reproductive health and rights. *Journal of the American Academy of Religion*, 73, 1155–1173.

O'Flaherty, M. and Fisher, J., 2008. Sexual orientation, gender identity and international human rights law: contextualising the Yogyakarta Principles. *Human Rights Law Review*, 8, 207–248.

Oxfam, 2010. Break another silence: understanding sexual minorities and taking action for sexual rights in Africa. Available from: http://publications.oxfam.org.uk/download.asp?dl=http://www.oxfam.org.uk/resources/policy/hivaids/downloads/break_another_silence_booklet.pdf [Accessed 20 Sept 2010].

Parsitau, D.S., 2009. Keep holy distance and abstain till he comes: interrogating a Pentecostal Church's engagements with HIV/AIDS and the youth in Kenya. *Africa Today*, 56, 45–64.

Perrin, K. and DeJoy, S.B., 2003. Abstinence-only education: how we got here and where we're going. *Journal of Public Health Policy*, 24, 445–459.

Pfeiffer, J., 2004. Condom social marketing, Pentecostalism, and structural adjustment in Mozambique: a clash of AIDS prevention messages. *Medical Anthropology Quarterly*, 18 (1), 77–103.

Phillips, O., 2004. (Dis)Continuities of custom in Zimbabwe and South Africa: the implications for gendered and sexual rights. *Health and Human Rights*, 7, 82–113.

PlusNews. 2011. Kenya: Catholics divided over Pope's condom comments. Available from: http://www.irinnews.org [Accessed 21 Jan 2011].

Pope Pius XII, 1951. Moral Questions Affecting Married Life. Addresses given 29 October 1951 to the Italian Catholic Union of midwives and 26 November 1951 to the National Congress of the Family Front and the Association of Large Families. Washington, DC: National Catholic Welfare Conference.

Prince, R., Denis, P., and van Dijk, T., 2009. Introduction to special issue: engaging Christianities: negotiating HIV/AIDS, health, and social relations in East and Southern Africa. *Africa Today*, 56, v–xviii.

Radio Vop Zimbabwe, 2010. No room for gay rights in new constitution-Mutasa. Available from: http://irma-rectalmicrobicides.blogspot.com/2010/06/zimbabwe-no-room-for-gay-rights-in-new.html [Accessed 1 Aug 2010].

Rankin, S.H., Lindgren, T., Kools, S.M., and Schell, E., 2008. The condom divide: disenfranchisement of Malawi women by church and state. *Journal of Obstetric, Gynecologic, & Neonatal Nursing*, 37, 596–606.

Rankin, S.H., Lindgren, T., Rankin, W.W., and Ng'oma, J., 2005. Donkey work: women, religion, and HIV/AIDS in Malawi. *Health Care for Women International*, 26, 4–16.

Sadgrove, J., 2007. Keeping up appearances: sex and religion amongst university students in Uganda. *Journal of Religion in Africa*, 37, 116–144.

Saiz, I., 2004. Bracketing sexuality: human rights and sexual orientation: a decade of development and denial at the UN. *Health and Human Rights*, 7, 48–80.

Santelli, J, Ott, M.A., Lyon, M., Rogers, J., Summers, D., and Schleifer, R., 2006. Abstinence and abstinence-only education: a review of U.S. policies and programs. *Journal of Adolescent Health*, 38, 72–81.

Schmid, B., 2006. AIDS discourses in the church: what we say and what we do. *Journal of Theology for Southern Africa*, 1, 91–103.

Senior, K., 2010. HIV, human rights, and men who have sex with men. *Lancet Infectious Diseases*, 10, 448–449.

Smith, D.J., 2004. Youth, sin and sex in Nigeria: Christianity and HIV/AIDS-related beliefs and behaviour among rural-urban migrants. *Culture, Health & Sexuality*, 6, 425–437.

Smith, S.M., 2009. Justification for human rights and the implications for HIV prevention. *Theology Today*, 66, 45–59.

South African Department of Health. 2007. *Medical Research Council, OrcMacro. South Africa Demographic and Health Survey 2003*. Pretoria: South Africa Department of Health.

Tharao, E., Massaqquoi, N., and Teclom, S., 2006. *Silent voices of the HIV/AIDS epidemic: African and Caribbean women in Toronto 2002–2004*. Toronto: Women's Health in Women's Hands Community Health Centre. Available from: http://www.whiwh.com [Accessed 3 Aug 2010].

Trinitapoli, J., 2006. Religious responses to AIDS in sub-Saharan Africa: an examination of religious congregations in rural Malawi. *Review of Religious Research*, 47, 253–270.

Trinitapoli, J., 2009. Religious teachings and influences on the ABCs of HIV prevention in Malawi. *Social Science & Medicine*, 69, 199–209.

Trinitapoli, J. and Regnerus, M.D., 2006. Religion and HIV risk behaviors among married men: initial results from a study in rural sub-Saharan Africa. *Journal for the Scientific Study of Religion*, 45, 505–528.

Twiss, S.B., 1998. Introduction to Roman Catholic perspectives on sexual orientation, human rights, and public policy. *In*: S.M. Olyan and M.C. Nussbaum, eds. *Sexual orientation & human rights in American religious discourse*. New York: Oxford University Press, 57–84.

Winfield, N., 2010. Vatican clarifies stance on condoms, birth control. *The Philadelphia Inquirer*, 22 December. Available from: http://www.edgeonthenet.com/index.php?ch=news&sc=&sc2=news&sc3=&id=114389 [Accessed 5 May 2011].

Wingood, G., 2010. Dissemination of HIV prevention interventions for women: collaborations with faith agencies & technological efforts. Available from: http://www.veomed.com/va041459962011 [Accessed 24 May 2010].

Yarber, S., 2010. Sexuality & the Bible. How do I read the Bible and why? Available from: http://mccgsl.org/#/sexuality-the-bible/4530903266 [Accessed 1 Oct 2010].

Civic/sanctuary orientation and HIV involvement among Chinese immigrant religious institutions in New York City

John J. Chin[a], Min Ying Li[a], Ezer Kang[b], Elana Behar[a] and Po Chun Chen[a]

[a]Department of Urban Affairs and Planning, Hunter College, City University of New York, New York, USA; [b]Department of Psychology, Wheaton College, Wheaton, Illinois, USA

Using data from a study of Chinese immigrant religious institutions in New York City (primarily Christian and Buddhist), this paper explores why some religious institutions are more inclined than others to be involved in HIV-related work. Although numerous factors are likely to play a role, we focus on organisations' differing views on social engagement as an explanatory factor. We hypothesise that religious institutions that value social engagement ('civic') will be more inclined towards HIV/AIDS involvement than those that are more inward focused ('sanctuary'). Given that many religious institutions are fundamentally defined by their stance on the appropriateness of social engagement, better understanding of this key characteristic may help to inform community and government organisations aiming to increase religious institutions' involvement in HIV/AIDS-related work. Our analysis suggests that some organisations may be less interested in taking on the challenges of working in HIV/AIDS because of their general view that churches or temples should not be socially engaged. On the other hand, religious institutions that have concerns about social acceptability, fear of infection or lack of capacity – but generally embrace social engagement – may be more open to partnering on HIV/AIDS-related work because of their overriding community service orientation.

Introduction

Religious organisations play key leadership roles in many communities and have the potential to be important participants in educating community members about HIV, supporting community members living with HIV and reducing HIV stigma. Indeed, some religious institutions have been very active in community HIV prevention efforts and in providing support and care to people living with HIV (Francis and Liverpool 2009, Derose et al. 2010b). However, religious institutions by and large have been reluctant to become involved in HIV-related activities, even in communities that have been particularly hard-hit by the AIDS epidemic (Cohen 1999, Genrich and Braithwaite 2005).

Using data from a study of Chinese immigrant religious institutions in New York City (NYC) – primarily Christian and Buddhist – this paper explores why some religious institutions are more inclined than others to be involved in

HIV-related work. Although numerous factors, such as perception of need, organisational capacity and social acceptability (Chin *et al.* 2005, Derose *et al.* 2010a), may influence a religious institutions' proclivity to participate in HIV-related work, we focus on organisations' differing institutional perspectives on the desirability of social engagement as an explanatory factor. We hypothesise that – even when they have concerns about social acceptability, fear of infection or lack of capacity – religious institutions with organisational cultures that value social engagement ('civic' organisations) will be more open to HIV/AIDS involvement than religious institutions that avoid social engagement ('sanctuary' organisations). In our analysis, we examine a range of organisational and member characteristics that may be related to a civic or a sanctuary orientation and then turn to analysing how a religious institution's civic or sanctuary orientation shapes its views on HIV involvement. Because religious institutions' stance on the appropriateness or desirability of social engagement is a fundamental, defining characteristic of many religious institutions (Dudley 1998), better understanding of this key characteristic may help to inform efforts to increase religious institutions' involvement in HIV/AIDS-related work.

Before delving into our analysis, we first provide an overview of Chinese immigrant religious institutions in NYC and HIV in Chinese immigrant communities and a discussion of the literature on religious institutions and social engagement.

Chinese immigrant religious institutions in NYC

There are numerous religious institutions in the Chinese immigrant community in NYC. In a previous study, we found that nearly half ($n = 132$) of the 316 NYC Chinese immigrant community institutions we identified were religious (Chin *et al.* 2005). In our current study, we identified 200 Chinese immigrant religious institutions in NYC's five boroughs (60.5% Christian, 29% Buddhist, and 10.5% Taoist and other religions).

In addition to being numerous, religious institutions are particularly influential due to the respect and trust they engender, their role in guiding values and behavioural norms (Kagimu *et al.* 1998), their tradition of community service, and their access to charitable resources and volunteers (Ross-Sheriff 2001). Their influence in immigrant communities is further augmented by members' reliance on them for everyday emotional and practical support, including counselling and even providing loans (Guest 2003, p. 129). The enormous influence of Asian immigrant religious institutions, coupled with their focus on behaviours that may be protective (Gray 2004, Hodge 2004), uniquely positions them to either confront the challenges of HIV or to maintain continued silence and stigmatisation regarding HIV in their communities. Constructive engagement with these institutions can foster the former role and, in the more extreme cases, at least mitigate any potential negative impact they have.

Chinese immigrants and HIV

The Chinese population in NYC is rapidly growing (Asian American Federation Census Information Center 2009) and is facing a changing HIV epidemic that may be affected by HIV/AIDS in China. In China, an estimated 740,000 people were living with HIV at the end of 2009, with an estimated 48,000 new infections in 2009 (Ministry of Health of the People's Republic of China 2010). In 2005, sexual transmission surpassed injection drug use as the main mode of transmission for *new* HIV cases in China. In some areas, 'HIV prevalence already exceeds 1% among pregnant women and those receiving premarital and clinical HIV testing, meeting UNAIDS criteria for generalized epidemic' (Ministry of Health of the People's Republic of China *et al.* 2006, p. 5). HIV transmission among men who have sex with men (MSM) constitutes a growing share of new HIV infections in China (32.5% of new cases in 2009) (Ministry of Health of the People's Republic of China 2010).

High levels of bi-directional migration between Asia and the USA suggest that the HIV epidemic in Asia has and will continue to affect Asians and Pacific Islanders (APIs) in the USA, including the Chinese-American population. For example, in a study of HIV-positive API immigrants in NYC, Chin *et al.* (2007b) found that several undocumented immigrant Chinese heterosexual men believed they were infected prior to entering the USA during long interim stays in Southeast Asia. A similar pattern was found in an HIV subtype analysis of a sample of individuals living with HIV in NYC, which included Chinese immigrant men who stopped in Burma or Thailand before arriving in the USA, during which time they reported having engaged in high-risk activity with female sex workers (Achkar *et al.* 2004).

In a review of HIV/AIDS data covering 2001 through 2004, the CDC found that APIs had the highest estimated annual percentage change in HIV/AIDS diagnosis rates in the USA (MMWR 2006, Chin *et al.* 2007a), suggesting a rapid increase in HIV/AIDS incidence. The NYC Department of Health and Mental Hygiene reported the same pattern for the same time period in NYC (NYCDOHMH 2006). Although these data suggest that rates of new HIV diagnoses are increasing among API women, transmission among MSM still accounted for the largest share of new HIV diagnoses among APIs in the USA (62.3%) and in NYC (51.4%) as of 2009 (NYCDOHMH 2010, Centers for Disease Control and Prevention 2011).

HIV/AIDS and associated behaviours, including extramarital sex, homosexuality and drug use, are highly stigmatised in API communities (Choi *et al.* 1995, Eckholdt *et al.* 1997, Sy *et al.* 1998, Chin and Kroesen 1999, Kang *et al.* 2000, Yoshikawa *et al.* 2001, Yoshioka and Schustack 2001). This stigmatisation has numerous consequences, including delays in HIV testing and care (Eckholdt and Chin 1997, Bhattacharya 2004), marginalisation and isolation of individuals living with HIV, resulting in poor mental health (Chin *et al.* 2007b) and lost opportunities for education regarding prevention and care (Kang *et al.* 2003). Compared to other populations in the USA, APIs have significantly lower rates of HIV testing, despite reporting similar rates of risk behaviour (Zaidi *et al.* 2005), and are uninformed about HIV, as there are few linguistically and culturally appropriate sources of information (Matteson 1997).

Religious institutions and social engagement

Many immigrant religious organisations are involved in providing a wide range of both formal and informal social services to immigrants, including orientation to the new country, housing and employment services, business opportunities, counselling, language classes and after-school programmes (Bankston and Zhou 2000, Cadge and Ecklund 2007, Foner and Alba 2008). Religious institution membership itself may provide immigrants with 'motivation, political information, and a space...to build communication and organizing skills' that are essential for civic engagement (Stoll and Wong 2007, p. 884). Overall, religious institutions may play a larger role than secular institutions in providing certain types of social services. For example, Botchwey (2007) found that, compared to secular institutions, a greater percentage of religious institutions in North Philadelphia were active in providing social, health and youth services.

Level of social engagement is often a fundamental defining characteristic of religious congregations (Dudley 1998, p. 125). A useful four-part typology to characterise churches' differing levels of societal engagement is provided by Roozen, McKinney and Carroll (Roozen *et al.* 1984):

- *Sanctuary:* generally uninvolved in the secular world; belief that good individual moral conduct will result in spiritual rewards after death.
- *Evangelical:* publicly engaged but for the purposes of propagating the religion rather than social change.
- *Civic:* strongly interested in public life; interested in working for social good through dominant social and political structures.
- *Activist:* also strongly interested in public life but more oriented towards social change and social justice than 'civic' congregations.

Failing to find a significant correlation between religious identity and social engagement, Mock (1992) re-organised the typology to separate these two dimensions. His religious identity dimension included 'evangelical', 'moderate' and 'liberal' to denote differing views on biblical literalism and the importance of the religious conversion experience. For the social engagement dimension, he kept the 'sanctuary', 'civic' and 'activist' categories, moving the 'evangelical' category to the religious identity dimension. Our paper uses the social engagement dimension of Mock's typology as a guide; we further reduce our social engagement categories to 'sanctuary' and 'civic' since none of the organisations in our sample were of the 'activist' type. Although the typology was developed for studying Christian churches, it applies well to our data on Buddhist temples.

Using data from a 1987 study of 'typical churches' in the mid-western USA, Mock (1992) identified key characteristics associated with differing levels of social engagement, including denomination, social views and church location. Although social engagement was more commonly found among mainline Protestant and Roman Catholic churches, civic and activist orientations were 'more common among conservative Protestant congregations than typically thought' (Mock 1992, p. 26), particularly in some Black and Hispanic congregations (Mock 1992, p. 22).[1]

In general, activist church members tended to be most liberal in their social views, and sanctuary church members tended to be most conservative, but this pattern varied (Mock 1992, p. 28). With regard to church location, 'more than 75% of the churches with an activist identity were located in inner city or inner city fringe neighbourhoods, as compared to 25% each for civic and sanctuary churches' (Mock 1992, p. 26). Mock (1992, p. 28) concludes that 'virtually any theological orientation can supply justification...for launching active, even radical, social ministry' (Mock 1992, p. 30).

Methods

Sampling and data collection

Data for this paper are from a five-year study on Chinese immigrant religious institutions and HIV involvement in NYC, funded by the US National Institutes of Health (Grant No. R01HD054303). To select institutions we first conducted a census of Chinese immigrant religious institutions in NYC, concentrating our efforts on three of NYC's five boroughs – Manhattan, Queens and Brooklyn – which have the largest Chinese populations and contain the three generally recognised Chinatowns of NYC. Institutions were first identified through published listings, Internet searches, and key informants and then by first-hand visual inspection of all the streets in census tracts with more than 1000 Chinese in 2000 and within a one-block radius of other known Chinese immigrant religious institutions. We then conducted a short survey with a random sample of 94 of the 200 religious institutions that we identified, and then randomly selected 21 organisations (11 Christian, 10 Buddhist) from the sample of 94 for in-depth study.

Within each of the 21 institutions, 8 religious leaders and active members were targeted for an in-depth qualitative interview. At the time this paper was written, 17 of the 21 institutions had been recruited, and 11 interviewers (3 full-time research associates and 8 part-time research assistants) had finished conducting 96 qualitative interviews (64 in Mandarin, 19 in Cantonese and 13 in English) between 60 and 90 minutes long. This paper relies primarily on an analysis of case studies developed using data from qualitative interviews and field notes from four organisations in our study.

Data management and analysis

Qualitative interviews were recorded using digital audio recorders and then translated and transcribed in English. The principal investigator, research associates and research consultants with expertise in theology, community psychology, HIV/ AIDS, immigrant populations and ethnographic research met three times as a committee to develop a codebook for coding the interviews. The initial codebook was based on the structure of the interview protocol and new themes that arose in the interviews. Each committee member used it to code the same interview to identify any problems or coding conflicts between coders. The codebook was then further refined, and each committee member then applied it to six additional interviews. The codebook was then further refined and finalised and then applied to the remaining interviews by a team of nine coders.

Based on the interviews and field notes, the Christian and Buddhist institutions were categorised as being of 'sanctuary' or 'civic' orientation based on their level of social engagement. Two Christian and two Buddhist institutions were identified as being particularly illustrative of the 'sanctuary' and 'civic' orientations and selected for case study development. In reporting our results below, we use pseudonyms to refer to the four case study organisations.

Results

Four case studies of Christian and Buddhist religious institutions with civic and sanctuary orientations

Community Welfare Church – civic, Christian

In our sample of Christian churches, seven were independent/non-denominational or evangelical churches, which tend to be more conservative, and only two were of mainline Protestant denominations. Both of the mainline Protestant churches in our sample fit the civic category. All of the evangelical/independent churches fit the sanctuary category, except for one – Community Welfare Church – which fit the civic category best. The profile of our church sample is consistent with Mock's finding that civic engagement is more commonly found among mainline Protestant churches but is not entirely absent in evangelical churches. We chose to develop our civic church case study around Community Welfare Church because, among the three civic churches, it embodied civic characteristics most strongly and also because it demonstrates that evangelical churches can be civically oriented.

Community Welfare Church, which is affiliated with a large Pentecostal denomination, was founded by an Indonesian-Chinese pastor. After a start in small home gatherings, the church settled into its current church building in Manhattan's Chinatown in 1978. Since then, Community Welfare Church has expanded to include a bilingual Sunday service attended by approximately 120 worshipers. The primarily ethnic-Chinese members vary widely in age and are originally from many different places, including Hong Kong, Taiwan and mainland China; there is also a substantial representation of ethnic-Chinese members born in Southeast Asian countries such as Malaysia and Indonesia. They work in a range of occupations, including civil servant, accountant and labourer, with sparser representation in elite professions like law and medicine. They live across the five boroughs of NYC with many commuting to Manhattan's Chinatown for worship services; only a small proportion of members come from outside of NYC. Diversity is evident in the church's decision-making body: members are from different age groups and professions, and both female and male. Diversity, church leaders and members say, is important to them because the church should accept a variety of viewpoints and work to 'break down all barriers of suspicion' among different groups. They also believe that diversity in leadership enhances the leadership's accountability to church members. Community Welfare Church leaders also believe in gender equality: 'we're equal in genders, we're equal in colours'.

Despite a general acceptance of diversity at the church, members have mixed feelings about homosexuality. For example, one member who works as a housekeeper for gay men found that her personal feelings towards her employers conflicted with her religious beliefs. She said:

> Initially, I looked down on them. However, once I got to know them well, I discovered they have very good hearts. When I told them that I was living in this country illegally, they helped me to obtain my legal status….They don't really harm us in any way. However, this is improper according to the Christian faith. Homosexuality is wrong.

In addition to holding regular religious events such as Sunday services and Bible study, the church also organises a wide range of local community activities and services, including a Chinese New Year Outreach; a block party; visits to nursing homes; provision of food for the homeless on Thanksgiving; a clothing drive for neighbourhood residents; and a one-week Vacation Bible School for young people to engage in arts, games, and of course 'a little bit of spiritual things'. Community Welfare Church is particularly interested in providing a safe haven for young people in the neighbourhood who congregate on the street after school because their immigrant parents work long hours and return home late in the evenings.

The church's annual block party in particular demonstrates Community Welfare Church's effort to reach out to the local Chinese community. The church started the block party five years ago to convey to the local community that 'our church is here' and 'there are certain things we can offer'. At the block party, the church distributes hotdogs, cotton candy and balloons, and each of the church's departments is responsible for giving a performance. In 2009, more than 300 people attended the block party, setting a new record for the church. Neighbourhood residents enjoy the food and entertainment and are encouraged to come to the church if they need help, such as assistance in reading and drafting English-language letters and forms.

Views on HIV involvement. Community Welfare Church's leaders and members are generally receptive to involvement in HIV-related work. Although church leaders and members expressed judgmental attitudes about HIV infection through 'sexual misconduct' as opposed to 'blood transfusion', they nevertheless felt that it was appropriate for the church to engage in HIV-related work, because 'if the church doesn't provide education, what other types of organisations would' and 'as Christians, [they] care for the sick'. Reflecting the church's mix of compassion and discomfort with HIV, one leader expressed an inflated concern about the infectiousness of HIV while also stating the need to remain caring: '[we] might be very cautious, but [we] have a very sympathetic heart'. After our first contact with them, leaders told us that they plan to distribute HIV educational materials at their next block party and asked us for sources of HIV educational pamphlets in Chinese and English.

These open and receptive attitudes may be influenced by the pastor, who had served as a minister to people with HIV in Malaysia. When he sensed that other congregants were unhappy about the presence of a sex worker and several drug users in attendance at his church, he approached each member individually and said, 'They are coming to be close to God. We have to support this, and we have to accept them'.

Queens Family Church – sanctuary, Christian

Queens Family church is located outside of the main Chinese enclaves in Queens (one of NYC's five boroughs), in a middle-class residential area. Affiliated with a large evangelical denomination that broke away from a mainline denomination, the church was founded in 1981 and serves both Cantonese- and English-speaking ethnic-Chinese members born in the USA, Hong Kong and mainland China. Most of the members live outside of the church's neighbourhood and commute to worship services; about half of the members commute in from outside of NYC's city limits, primarily from Long Island and New Jersey. Membership at Queens Family Church is made up of predominantly middle-class professionals, with many families with young children.

Although gender equality is commonly emphasised by leaders and members of Queens Family Church, a number of men as well as women in the church believe that a woman's role is to support men's decisions, and men are chiefly responsible for deciding church matters. This has resulted in harboured negative feelings among some women at the church and has resulted in the loss of some members. As one female member explained: 'Many times [I wanted to leave the church]. Sometimes my own opinion was not taken….I said to myself, this is not what I want to be in'. Regarding homosexuality, Queens Family Church leaders and members somewhat uniformly perceive homosexuality as 'just like any other sin', including ones as extreme as murder, and believe that homosexuality is 'against God's design'.

Since young families are one of the largest groups in Queens Family Church, many church programmes target children, including an afterschool programme, a Chinese school, and a Summer Vacation Bible school. For adult and elderly members, the church has organised vocational assistance and health seminars. However, these services have had only limited success, partly because of the church's location, reflecting Mock's (1992) finding of lower levels of social engagement outside of inner city areas. For example, although the Chinese school is a free service for neighbourhood and members' children, attendance is low because parents have other priorities for their children, such as SAT prep classes. According to the church's pastor, 'if we were in a poor community, it might be easier because the kids would need somebody to care for them'. The church has also had limited success with its afterschool programmes and health seminars. As a lay leader explains, 'I guess [these programmes aren't successful] because we are not in Flushing [Chinese neighbourhood in Queens]….Also, I guess this neighbourhood is more middle-class, and people don't look to come to church to learn about health matters'.

Unlike its work in the local Chinese community, the church's work in international and domestic charity is more successful. Fundraising to respond to natural disasters overseas and in the USA occurs regularly at the church. The church, for example, has collected second-hand eyeglasses and cell phones to donate to developing countries and has financially assisted a school in Thailand. Most recently, they organised a clothing drive for Haiti, and one of their members was part of a Christian group providing free medical care in Haiti.

Views on HIV involvement. In keeping with many churches' view that caring for the ill is an important form of Christian service, the leaders at Queens Family Church expressed compassion towards people with HIV. Leaders at Queens Family Church also agreed that community members lack HIV awareness possibly because HIV is a taboo subject in Chinese communities. However, in contrast to the leaders at Community Welfare Church, leaders at Queens Family Church are reluctant to get involved in HIV-related efforts. Leaders had concerns about the church's image, the stigma that members might experience because of the church's HIV involvement, and the potential conflict between their religious teachings and the contents of HIV educational efforts. Finally, there was a perception that members were not in need of HIV education because their Christian training would be sufficient protection against HIV risk. One prominent member, the wife of the senior pastor, said, 'HIV education isn't really necessary here because no one here has HIV. In fact, you will find that Christians do not have HIV…'.

Temple of Engaged Buddhism – civic, Buddhist

Established in 1979 and one of the oldest temples in Manhattan's Chinatown, the Temple of Engaged Buddhism was founded in part to provide immigrants with a place where they could feel they belonged while adjusting to life in a new country. Engaged Buddhism Temple has about 50 members participating in a weekly Sunday Dharma service, over 800 participants on religious holidays, and over 3000 on Lunar New Year. When Engaged Buddhism Temple hosted their 30th anniversary celebration banquet to fundraise for construction of a temple in upstate New York, 1000 tickets were sold.

As at many Chinese Buddhist temples in NYC's Chinatowns, members of Engaged Buddhism Temple tend to be older adults and mostly working class. Typical member occupations include housekeeper, home attendant and restaurant worker. A number of members were born in Hong Kong and China, and there is a substantial presence of ethnic-Chinese from Southeast Asian countries, including Malaysia and Burma. Many members are from the local Chinatown community; others travel in from Brooklyn or Queens, but almost no members come from outside of NYC.

Although the head of the temple, the abbot, is male, leaders at Engaged Buddhism Temple believe that women and men are equal, and women hold important temple leadership positions. As one leader explained:

> It's not because I am a man, therefore I should stand taller than you. Or because I am a woman, I should deserve more services.... The same set of rules should be applied to both genders.... Simply because I go to work all day doesn't make me any more important. Or if you stay home and cook, that doesn't mean you should be more obedient. These things are not applicable nowadays. Both men and women are part of today's workforce.

Regarding homosexuality, temple members expressed mixed feelings. While some members perceived homosexuality as 'abnormal and immoral', others perceived it as a private matter: 'this is purely a personal matter related to a sexual act. This is no big deal'.

Many activities at Engaged Buddhism Temple are primarily religious, including the weekly Dharma service and participation in a parade honouring Buddha's birthday. However, Engaged Buddhism Temple is also actively engaged in secular community activities. For example, the temple organised a health fair in 2008 to provide basic health education, blood pressure screening and diabetes testing. Supportive counselling is also provided to members on an as-needed basis, although counselling is mostly delivered in the context of Buddhist teachings and philosophies. Engaged Buddhism Temple also tried to establish a Chinese school, although the effort ended a few years ago due to limited space and human resources.

Views on HIV involvement. The Temple of Engaged Buddhism is one of the few Chinese religious organisations in our study that has been involved in HIV education activities. Although leaders at Engaged Buddhism Temple said they believed that Buddhist precepts are sufficient to guide people's behaviours and to prevent HIV infection, they still agreed to host an HIV education workshop conducted by a community organisation at the temple. The workshop covered a wide range of HIV-related topics, including topics considered taboo by many Chinese Buddhists – such as sex and homosexuality. Some of the temple's religious leaders attended the workshop, including the abbot himself. Later the abbot said that he thought it was appropriate and important for the temple to educate community members about HIV and that all of the temple's members would support such an effort. Even so, he expressed concerns about capacity: 'we don't have the capability and we don't know how to do those activities, but if outside people were to do them here, we would be absolutely supportive and cooperative'.

Refuge Buddhist Temple – sanctuary, Buddhist

Refuge Buddhist Temple was founded by a successful Chinese-American entrepreneur and a high monk from mainland China in the 1960s. Unlike the Temple of Engaged Buddhism, which is centrally located in Manhattan's Chinatown, Refuge Buddhist Temple is located in one of N Y C's outer boroughs, far from any Chinese ethnic enclave. Most of the members are Mandarin-speaking middle-class professionals or home-makers from Taiwan who currently live in the metropolitan New York area away from the temple's neighbourhood. More than half of the members travel in from outside of NYC, from New Jersey, Long Island and upstate New York. Refuge Buddhist Temple, in contrast to Temple of Engaged Buddhism, has Dharma services only twice a month rather than weekly. Small-group, informal Buddhist reading clubs are organised among members closer to their homes. The temple's religious leaders periodically travel to different towns or neighbourhoods in the metropolitan area to teach Buddhism at the reading clubs. For religious holidays, about 50–60 people attend ceremonies at the temple.

Interestingly, Refuge Buddhist Temple is run almost entirely by women (an abbess and nuns), complicating the notion that inclusion of women in the leadership is associated with a civic orientation. Moreover, members' views on gender equality tend to be similar to those of organisations with a civic orientation, for example: 'Nowadays women can have a lot of power, can have a lot of responsibilities..., so the genders should be equal'. For an organisation that is run by women and attended mostly by women, however, views on gender are surprisingly mixed. For example, another member said:

> ...Everyone has his/her own role in this society. Women are to bear children and take care of children; men are to go out to work and support families. Women can help to support their families now; men can also help...But the important thing is how do you bear children? It's just not possible for men, right?

Similarly to the Temple of Engaged Buddhism, Refuge Buddhist Temple also expressed mixed views about homosexuality. Some members felt that homosexuality is 'against nature', while other members believed that homosexuality is acceptable, particularly when it remains a private matter. Unlike at the Temple of Engaged Buddhism, however, no interviewees at Refuge Buddhist Temple expressed unequivocal acceptance of homosexuality.

Refuge Buddhist Temple's general 'sanctuary' orientation appears to pervade the efforts the temple has made to interact more with the local community. Since the temple is not located in a Chinese community, leaders have considered opening a facility for English-speaking neighbourhood residents. They have not taken any action in this direction, however, because of concerns about safety and language barriers. Their safety fears are based partly on negative racial stereotypes. As the abbess said: 'I personally worry about safety issues, since we're all women here. Before we didn't prevent anyone from coming in, but then we discovered the "merit box" [donation box] was taken. There are a lot of Blacks here, so I have to think about safety issues'. The statement unfortunately reflects racial prejudice at the temple and a reluctance to work through those prejudices to bridge differences.

Views on HIV involvement. HIV is a controversial issue at Refuge Buddhist Temple. Although several interviewees stated that it is appropriate for Refuge Buddhist Temple to be involved in HIV-related work because of religious mandates concerning compassion, they were reluctant to get involved, partly because of their fears of HIV infection through casual contact. They also felt that it would be difficult for them to extend care to persons living with HIV because of their limited HIV knowledge. Leaders also said that they would be more inclined to help a person who became infected with HIV through a blood transfusion but would not extend themselves to help a person who became infected through 'immoral' behaviour (e.g., sexual behaviour). The treatment of a nun at the temple with Hepatitis C (infected through a blood transfusion) suggests that fear of infection and stigma might prevent an accepting response to any person with HIV. In one interview, a leader described how this nun has been assigned a separate bedroom, bathroom and kitchen because of her illness.

Similar to Queens Family Church (the 'sanctuary' church), Refuge Buddhist Temple perceives HIV as a disease for 'socially and culturally lower' classes. Accordingly, they feel that members of the temple do not need HIV education 'since the standards of the members are high and their incomes levels are high'; in contrast, they believe that Chinese in Chinatown, new immigrants and young people may need HIV education.

Discussion

In discussing the four case studies, we aim to draw links between organisational characteristics and their civic or sanctuary orientation. To highlight patterns, Table 1 below organises the organisational and member characteristics discussed in the case studies above by civic and sanctuary orientation. Table 1 is then followed by a discussion that analyses resulting patterns and draws out the implications of civic or sanctuary orientations for organisational involvement in HIV. Because our qualitative, case study sample of respondents is relatively small and not randomly selected, our findings may not be representative and cannot be generalised to the larger Chinese immigrant religious community. The next phases of our research will use quantitative instruments with a larger, randomly selected sample to produce more generalisable findings. The richness of qualitative case studies, however, provides insights that quantitative research often cannot.

Comparing civic and sanctuary institutions

A review of Table 1 suggests that, compared to sanctuary organisations, civic organisations are more likely to be located in an ethnic enclave; to have a

Table 1. Organisational and member characteristics by civic/sanctuary orientation.

	Civic	Sanctuary
Location	In Chinese ethnic enclave	Outside of Chinese ethnic enclave
Member residence	Primarily within New York City	Half or more outside of NYC (upstate New York, Long Island and New Jersey)
Member socio-economic status	Wide range of occupations with substantial representation in working class jobs	Large proportion of middle class home-makers and white-collar professionals
Member ethnic backgrounds	Substantial representation of ethnic-Chinese from Southeast Asia (Malaysia, Burma, Vietnam and Indonesia)	Primarily from Mainland China, Hong Kong and Taiwan
Diversity of leadership	Leadership and decision-making bodies are diverse (e.g., age, occupation, gender)	Leadership and decision-making bodies are dominated by either men (church) or women (temple)
Views on gender equality and diversity	Leaders embrace gender equality and diversity of membership and leadership	Leaders have mixed views on gender equality and have concerns about introducing diversity into the membership and leadership
Views on homosexuality	Mixed views, with some members expressing unequivocal acceptance	Uniform condemnation of homosexuality (church) and mixed views (temple)

membership that resides primarily within NYC's limits and is more working class and ethnically diverse; and to have greater age, occupational and gender diversity represented in the leadership. Civic organisations were also more accepting of gender equality, diversity and homosexuality. The patterns were remarkably consistent within the civic and sanctuary categories even when comparing across religions. In other words, the civic Buddhist temple and the civic Christian church in many ways resembled each other more than they did the sanctuary organisations of their own religion. The differing stances on social engagement of the two Christian churches – both affiliated with conservative evangelical denominations – also suggest that religious denomination is not necessarily defining of an organisation's civic/sanctuary orientation.

The civic organisations' greater ability to fulfil a civic mission may be largely determined by the physical location of the institutions. Community Welfare Church and Temple of Engaged Buddhism are in touch with community members with a variety of needs because of their physical location in Manhattan's Chinatown, while Queens Family Church and Refuge Buddhist Temple are more removed from the Chinese community, therefore not having the same chance to provide community services. This pattern is consistent with Botchwey's (2007) finding that religious organisations that have remained in inner city areas are knowledgeable of local residents needs and committed to addressing them. Awareness of local needs may also be facilitated in the civic organisations by the fact that most members live in the local area or at least within NYC's limits.

Comparing the locations of the organisations begs the question of whether they chose their locations to correspond to their civic/sanctuary orientation or whether their civic/sanctuary orientations were shaped by their locations. This question is unanswerable in this study, but worthy of future research. The organisations' histories at least show that the civic church and temple have never been located in a Chinatown and that the sanctuary church and temple have never been located outside of a Chinatown.

The civic church and temple may also be more receptive to working more closely with the community because of their memberships' and leaderships' greater diversity (e.g., in terms of socio-economic class, country of origin, and a balance between men and women in the leadership). The experience of diversity may make the civic organisations more aware of community concerns, more accepting of people who are different and more open to new ideas, in contrast to the sanctuary organisations, where a greater homogeneity among members may perpetuate discomfort with difference and pressure to conform. As with the question of location noted above, however, the causal direction cannot be determined with our data.

The case studies suggest that wealthier religious organisations in Chinese immigrant communities may be more socially conservative than less wealthy ones. Wealthier immigrants, having few needs themselves, may feel insulated from the concerns of poorer immigrants and may in fact seek out churches that provide a refuge from worldly concerns. According to Yang (1998), conservative ethnic churches provide an absolute biblical ethos that is valued by immigrants as they face the uncertainties of modernity in a new country. Organisational wealth may also make a congregation less dependent on the surrounding community. Community Welfare Church, for example, tries to engage the community to increase membership, and thereby contributions, and to raise money through leasing their space. Queens Family Church's wealthier membership, in contrast, makes such money-raising activities less necessary. Taking on issues that threaten to alienate current members could be detrimental to a religious organisation's member-based wealth, a situation that may discourage the kind of bold, new initiative that HIV involvement would represent in most Chinese immigrant churches and temples.

Civic/sanctuary orientation and HIV involvement

The previous discussion explores various organisational and membership characteristics that might help to predict or identify civic or sanctuary orientation. We now turn to examining the relationship between civic/sanctuary orientation and the likelihood and probable forms of organisational involvement in HIV-related efforts. Unlike the sanctuary institutions, the civic church and temple readily indicated willingness to be involved in HIV-related efforts. The civic church was proactive in asking about how to acquire HIV education brochures and planned to distribute those brochures at its next block party. Similarly, the civic Buddhist temple actually hosted an HIV education workshop at the temple. Although misinformed fears of HIV infection and judgmental attitudes towards those infected with HIV through sex were evident to some degree in all four case studies, these concerns appeared to be less significant barriers to HIV involvement for civically oriented institutions.

Although both civic and sanctuary institutions expressed compassion for people living with HIV, the civic church, in particular, explicitly expressed acceptance of stigmatised groups often associated with HIV (e.g., sex workers, drug users). Views on homosexuality in the civic institutions ranged from mixed to full acceptance; whereas views in the sanctuary institutions ranged from mixed to full condemnation. Regarding the role of religion type, it is noteworthy that views on homosexuality in the Buddhist temples were informed far less by religious doctrine than in the churches, where accepting views of homosexuality were limited by most interviewees' belief that the Bible clearly condemns homosexuality. This pattern is consistent with Detenber *et al.*'s (2007) finding in Singapore that Christians held more negative attitudes towards homosexuality than Buddhists, whose core religious texts do not discuss homosexuality. Religious organisations' views on homosexuality – as well as on gender equality – are important to consider since these views may limit the range of sexual activities and prevention strategies that they might be willing to address. These views may also determine whether their messages about sexual orientation and gender equality are empowering or further stigmatising. Prevention efforts that fail to non-judgmentally address community members' specific risk behaviours or that promote stigma or inequality may be counter-productive.

The various characteristics associated with civically oriented churches and temples may be helpful in identifying more willing partners for HIV-related efforts that take a more empowering and less judgmental approach. We should, however, take note of Mock's (1992) challenge to avoid narrow interpretations of religious typologies. Mock found that the assumed linear relationship between a 'congregation's...religious style and its involvement in society...is more mythical than real' (Mock 1992, p. 22). In our study sample, for instance, one of the most accepting institutions with regard to HIV was Community Welfare Church, an evangelical church affiliated with a very conservative denomination. Although we excluded religious identity from the typology reflected in Table 1, Mock's caution is still warranted given that overly relying on any typology may unnecessarily narrow our expectations of an institution's potential for involvement in HIV-related work.

Avoiding potential partnerships simply because they may pose some challenges may result in excluding religious organisations that could be important contributors or reach communities that would not otherwise be reached. Rather than use typologies to predict whether an institution will engage in HIV-related work, we might use them to consider how best to approach institutions and also to assess their potential strengths and weaknesses. Finding ways to include a wider range of religious institutions to participate constructively in HIV-related efforts will ensure that a broader swath of community members is reached with information and support.

Acknowledgements

Research for this article was supported by a grant from the National Institute of Child Health and Human Development (Grant No. R01HD054303). The authors received valuable feedback when a version of this work was presented at the Conference on HIV/AIDS and Religious Cultures and Institutions, held at Columbia University, Mailman School of Public Health, 12 July 2010. The authors would like to thank the Editor and anonymous reviewers for their helpful comments. We are also grateful to leaders and members of participating religious institutions who generously shared their time and stories.

Note

1. The role of the church as an 'organizational and psychological resource for individual and collective political action' in African-American communities is also explored by Harris (1994). Morris' (1984) seminal work on the civil rights movement also documents the key role of Black churches in enabling the movement.

References

Achkar, J.M., Burda, S.T., Konings, F.A., Urbanski, M.M., Williams, C.A., Seifen, D., Kahirimbanyi, M.N., Vogler, M., Parta, M., Lupatkin, H.C., Zolla-Pazner, S., and Nyambi, P.N., 2004. Infection with HIV type 1 group m non-b subtypes in individuals living in New York City. *Journal of Acquired Immune Deficiency Syndrome*, 36 (3), 835–844.

Asian American Federation Census Information Center, 2009. *Profile of New York City's Chinese Americans: 2005–2007*. New York: Asian American Federation of New York. Available from: http://www.aafny.org/cic/briefs/chinese2009.pdf [Accessed date 29 October 2010].

Bankston, C.L. and Zhou, M., 2000. De facto congregationalism and socioeconomic mobility in Laotian and Vietnamese immigrant communities: a study of religious institutions and economic change. *Review of Religious Research*, 41, 453–470.

Bhattacharya, G., 2004. Health care seeking for HIV/AIDS among South Asians in the United States. *Health and Social Work*, 29 (2), 106–115.

Botchwey, N.D., 2007. The religious sector's presence in local community development. *Journal of Planning Education and Research*, 27 (1), 36–48.

Cadge, W. and Ecklund, E.H., 2007. Immigration and religion. *Annual Review of Sociology*, 33, 259–379.

Centers for Disease Control and Prevention (CDC), 2011. *HIV surveillance report, 2009, 21*. Atlanta: Centers for Disease Control and Prevention. Available from: http://www.cdc.gov/hiv/topics/surveillance/resources/reports/.

Chin, D. and Kroesen, K.W., 1999. Disclosure of HIV infection among Asian/Pacific Islander American women: cultural stigma and social support. *Cultural Diversity and Ethnic Minority Psychology*, 5 (3), 222–235.

Chin, J.J., Leung, M., Sheth, L., and Rodriguez, T.R., 2007a. Let's not ignore a growing HIV problem for Asians and Pacific Islanders in the U.S. *Journal of Urban Health*, 84 (5), 642–647.

Chin, J.J., Mantell, J., Weiss, L., Bhagavan, M., and Luo, X., 2005. Chinese and South Asian religious institutions and HIV prevention in New York City. *AIDS Education & Prevention*, 17 (5), 484–502.

Chin, J.J., Weiss, L., Kang, E., Abramson, D., Bartlett, N., Behar, E., and Aidala, A., 2007b. *Looking for a place to call home: a needs assessment of Asians and Pacific Islanders living with HIV/AIDS in the New York eligible metropolitan area*. New York: The New York Academy of Medicine.

Choi, K.H., Coates, T.J., Catania, J.A., Lew, S., and Chow, P., 1995. High HIV risk among gay Asian and Pacific Islander men in San Francisco. *AIDS*, 9 (3), 306–308.

Cohen, C.J., 1999. *The boundaries of blackness: AIDS and the breakdown of black politics*. Chicago: University of Chicago Press.

Derose, K.P., Mendel, P.J., Kanouse, D.E., Bluthenthal, R.N., Castaneda, L.W., Hawes-Dawson, J., Mata, M., and Oden, C.W., 2010a. Learning about urban congregations and HIV/AIDS: community-based foundations for developing congregational health interventions. *Journal of Urban Health*, 87 (4), 617–630.

Derose, K.P., Mendel, P.J., Palar, K., Kanouse, D.E., Bluthenthal, R.N., Castaneda, L.W., Corbin, D.E., Dominguez, B.X., Hawes-Dawson, J., Mata, M.A., and Oden, C.W., 2010b. Religious congregations' involvement in HIV: a case study approach. *AIDS and Behavior* [online first edition]. Available from: http://www.springerlink.com/content/gv28532384235620/ [Accessed 19 October 2010].

Detenber, B.H., Cenite, M., Ku, M.K.Y., Ong, C.P.L., Tong, H.Y., and Yeow, M.L.H., 2007. Singaporeans' attitudes toward lesbians and gay men and their tolerance of media portrayals of homosexuality. *International Journal of Public Opinion Research*, 19 (3), 367–379.

Dudley, C.S., 1998. Process: dynamics of congregational life. *In*: N.T. Ammerman, J.W. Carroll, C.S. Dudley, and W. Mckinney, eds. *Studying congregations*. Nashville: Abingdon Press, 105–131.

Eckholdt, H. and Chin, J., 1997. Pneumocystis carinii pneumonia in Asians and Pacific Islanders. *Clinical Infectious Diseases*, 24 (6), 1265–1267.

Eckholdt, H.M., Chin, J.J., Manzon-Santos, J.A., and Kim, D.D., 1997. The needs of Asians and Pacific Islanders living with HIV in New York City. *AIDS Education & Prevention*, 9 (6), 493–504.

Foner, N. and Alba, R., 2008. Immigrant religion in the US and Western Europe: bridge or barrier to inclusion? *International Migration Review*, 42 (2), 360–392.

Francis, S.A. and Liverpool, J., 2009. A review of faith-based HIV prevention programs. *Journal of Religion and Health*, 48 (1), 6–15.

Genrich, G.L. and Braithwaite, B.A., 2005. Response of religious groups to HIV/AIDS as a sexually transmitted infection in Trinidad. *BMC Public Health*, 5, 1–12.

Gray, P.B., 2004. HIV and Islam: is HIV prevalence lower among Muslims. *Social Science & Medicine*, 58, 1751–1756.

Guest, K.J., 2003. *God in Chinatown: religion and survival in New York's evolving immigrant community*. New York: New York University Press.

Harris, F.C., 1994. Something within: religion as a mobilizer of African-American political activism. *The Journal of Politics*, 56 (1), 42–68.

Hodge, D.R., 2004. Working with Hindu clients in a spiritually sensitive manner. *Social Work*, 49 (1), 27–38.

Kagimu, M., Marum, E., Wabwire-Mangen, F., Nakyanjo, N., Walakira, Y., and Hogle, J., 1998. Evaluation of the effectiveness of AIDS health education interventions in the Muslim community in Uganda. *AIDS Education & Prevention*, 10 (3), 215–228.

Kang, E., Rapkin, B.D., Kim, J.H., Springer, C., and Chhabra, R., 2000. *Voices: an assessment of needs among Asian and Pacific Islander undocumented non-citizens living with HIV disease in New York City*. New York: Mayor's Office of AIDS Policy Coordination and the New York HIV Health and Human Services Planning Council.

Kang, E., Rapkin, B.D., Springer, C., and Kim, J.H., 2003. The 'Demon plague' and access to care among Asian undocumented immigrants living with HIV disease in New York City. *Journal of Immigrant Health*, 5 (2), 49–58.

Matteson, D.R., 1997. Bisexual and homosexual behavior and HIV risk among Chinese-, Filipino-, and Korean-American men. *Journal of Sex Research*, 34 (1), 93–104.

Ministry of Health of the People's Republic of China, 2010. *China 2010 UNGASS country progress report (2008–2009)*. Beijing: Ministry of Health of the People's Republic of China.

Ministry of Health of the People's Republic of China, UNAIDS & World Health Organization, 2006. *2005 update on the HIV/AIDS epidemic and response in China*. Beijing: National Center for AIDS/STD Prevention and Control, China CDC.

MMWR, 2006. Racial/ethnic disparities in diagnoses of HIV/AIDS–33 states, 2001–2004. *MMWR Morbidity and Mortal Weekly Report*, 55 (5), 121–125.

Mock, A.K., 1992. Congregational religious styles and orientations to society: exploring our linear assumptions. *Review of Religious Research*, 34 (1), 20–33.

Morris, A.D., 1984. *The origins of the civil rights movement: black communities organizing for change*. New York: The Free Press.

NYCDOHMH, 2006. *HIV/AIDS in New York City, 2001–2004*. New York: New York City Department of Health and Mental Hygiene.

NYCDOHMH, 2010. New York City HIV/AIDS annual surveillance statistics. New York: New York City Department of Health and Mental Hygiene.

Roozen, D.A., Mckinney, W., and Carroll, J.W., 1984. *Varieties of religious presence*. New York: Pilgrim Press.

Ross-Sheriff, F., 2001. Immigrant Muslim women in the United States: adaptation to American society. *Journal of Social Work Research*, 2 (2), 283–294.

Stoll, M.A. and Wong, J.S., 2007. Immigration and civic participation in a multiracial and multiethnic context. *International Migration Review*, 41 (4), 880–908.

Sy, F.S., Chng, C.L., Choi, S.T., and Wong, F.Y., 1998. Epidemiology of HIV and AIDS among Asian and Pacific Islander Americans. *AIDS Education & Prevention*, 10 (3 Suppl), 4–18.

Yang, F., 1998. Chinese conversion to evangelical Christianity: the importance of social and cultural contexts. *Sociology of Religion*, 59 (3), 237–257.

Yoshikawa, H., Wilson, P., Hsueh, J., Rosman, E.A., Chin, J., and Kim, J.H., 2001. What front-line NGO staff can tell us about culturally anchored theories of change in HIV prevention for Asian/Pacific Islanders in the U.S. *American Journal of Community Psychology*, 32 (1–2), 143–158.

Yoshioka, M.R. and Schustack, A., 2001. Disclosure of HIV status: cultural issues of Asian patients. *AIDS Patient Care & STDs*, 15 (2), 77–82.

Zaidi, I.F., Crepaz, N., Song, R., Wan, C.K., Lin, L.S., Hu, D.J., and Sy, F.S., 2005. Epidemiology of HIV/AIDS among Asians and Pacific Islanders in the United States. *AIDS Education and Prevention*, 17 (5), 405–417.

Ideologies of Black churches in New York City and the public health crisis of HIV among Black men who have sex with men

Patrick A. Wilson, Natalie M. Wittlin, Miguel Muñoz-Laboy and Richard Parker

Department of Sociomedical Sciences, Columbia University, New York, NY, USA

Black men who have sex with men (MSM) are disproportionately affected by HIV and AIDS in New York City (NYC). Black churches in NYC have a history of engaging in community mobilisation; however, research suggests that churches play a role in promoting stigma against Black MSM, which impedes prevention efforts. The goal of this study was to explore church ideologies surrounding sexuality and health, and the relationship of these ideologies to church mobilisation in response to HIV/AIDS among Black MSM. We conducted interviews and focus groups with pastors and parishioners at Black churches in NYC. Three prominent themes were identified: (1) 'Love the sinner, hate the sin' – distinguishing behaviour and identity; (2) 'Don't ask, don't tell' – keeping same-sex behaviour private; and (3) 'Your body is a temple' – connecting physical and spiritual health. We discuss the implications of these ideologies for church mobilisation and HIV prevention efforts. In doing so, we pay close attention to how ideologies may both impede and facilitate church dialogue around sexuality and heightened responses to the HIV crisis affecting Black MSM.

Introduction

Black churches in the USA play an important role in the culture and social lives of many Black Americans (Lincoln and Mamiya 1990, Taylor *et al.* 1999). While Black communities and individuals vary in the extent to which they are directly involved with churches, Black churches remain a strong force in the lives of Black Americans. A recent Pew Forum (2008) survey of the US religious landscape found that of all racial/ethnic groups in the USA, Black Americans were the most likely to report being affiliated with a religious institution; 85% of Black Americans reported a Christian affiliation. Even among Black Americans who reported being religiously unaffiliated, three in four said that religion was either somewhat or very important in their lives (compared to just above one in three of the overall unaffiliated population).

Black churches and community mobilisation

Many Black churches have historically been involved in social and political movements, the most commonly cited example being the Civil Rights Movement of the 1950s and 1960s. Then and now, churches have helped to mobilise Black communities around pressing social and health issues, thereby facilitating positive change (Lincoln and Mamiya 1990). Scholars have theorised about and debated the mechanisms by which Black churches enable – or fail to enable – mobilisation around social and health issues (Pattillo-McCoy 1998, Harris 1999, Barnes 2005, McClerking and McDaniel 2005). While research has tended to focus on 'church culture' (i.e., common rituals and practices) rather than religious ideology, it has also considered the commonly held belief that God is active in worldly affairs (Pattillo-McCoy 1998). This work suggests that a unique relationship between culture and theology exists in many Black churches. Harris (1999) articulates this relationship, noting that Black church-based social movements have benefited from a 'sacred assurance', or the feeling that actions are validated by scripture and that God is on the side of the church. This sense of sacred assurance, Harris notes, has promoted feelings of personal and collective efficacy among Black Christians involved in church mobilisation efforts. Other researchers have pointed to a number of specific factors and activities that affect church mobilisation including: dialogue and information-sharing among parishioners (McKenzie 2004); prayer groups and gospel music (Barnes 2005); cost-underwriting and obligation-creating activities (McClerking and McDaniel 2005); and a 'tool kit' that includes prayer, call-and-response, verbal encouragement, Christian imagery and a sense of 'collective ethos' (Pattillo-McCoy 1998). Recent Black church community mobilisation efforts have focused on a variety of public health issues including care for older adults (Madison and McGadney 2000), prison reintegration (O'Connor et al. 1998) and breast and cervical cancer (Shapiro et al. 2006), among others.

Black churches in New York City (NYC) – the setting of our research study – have played a particularly prominent role in community mobilisation efforts focused on social issues, historically and contemporarily (Bunche 1973). In the 1920s and 1930s, the social gospel movement flourished in Black communities, and social justice-oriented religious leaders such as Adam Clayton Powell, Sr., Reverdy Ransom, and Shelton Hale Bishop used churches as spaces for social service and action (Spencer 1996). Black churches in NYC have also made efforts to mobilise the community to prevent HIV/AIDS since the beginning of the epidemic. As reported by Quimby and Friedman (2003), Black churches in NYC began to mobilise against HIV/AIDS in late 1987, organising community forums and educational conferences held at various churches, including the historic Concord Baptist Church in Brooklyn. Contemporarily, Black churches in NYC are still involved in community responses to HIV/AIDS. For example, the current pastor of Abyssinian Baptist, Dr. Calvin O. Butts, III, sits on the Presidential Advisory Commission on HIV/AIDS (PACHA) and leads the National Black Leadership Commission on AIDS (United States Department of Health and Human Services [DHHS] 2010). Black churches in NYC have demonstrated leadership in promoting awareness and mobilisation around issues affecting the communities they serve.

Stigma and responses to HIV/AIDS among Black churches

Stigma surrounding HIV, homosexuality and behaviours associated with HIV transmission have historically impeded Black church mobilisation in response to HIV/AIDS (Fullilove and Fullilove 1999, Quimby and Friedman 2003). Research suggests that associations between HIV/AIDS and homosexuality have hindered Black churches' responses to the HIV/AIDS crisis affecting Black men who have sex with men (MSM). Black churches have often been sources of homophobia and heterosexism in the lives of Black MSM (Miller 2007, Harris 2009), and perceived associations between HIV/AIDS, homosexuality and White communities may impede their responses to the epidemic (Nelson 2005).

In the past few years, however, researchers have documented efforts at HIV prevention, education and stigma reduction in churches and faith communities. For example, a faith-based intervention that aimed to increase HIV/AIDS awareness and decrease HIV stigma gained traction in a Black faith community in Michigan (Griffith et al. 2010). Also, a recent qualitative study of 14 Northeast churches with HIV/AIDS programming found that lay health leaders were organising both educational activities and testing events and that these leaders recognised barriers to prevention work, such as stigma, within the context of their churches. Results from the study suggested that a 'fundamental change in how Black churches are approaching HIV/AIDS in the Black community' is underway and that 'churches appear to be fertile ground for prevention work' (Davis 2008).

The need for community-level responses from Black churches

The current study aimed to explore NYC-based churches' ideologies surrounding sexuality, health and HIV/AIDS, as well as how these ideologies relate to church mobilisation in response to the HIV/AIDS epidemic among Black MSM. HIV/AIDS among Black MSM is a public health crisis that has not been adequately addressed in the USA (White House Office of National AIDS Policy 2010). Black MSM are disproportionately affected by HIV/AIDS in the USA and continue to experience a rapidly increasing HIV incidence. A recently conducted epidemiological study of 8153 MSM in 21 US cities found that 28% of non-Hispanic Black MSM were infected with HIV, the highest prevalence among all ethnic/racial groups examined (Centers for Disease Control and Prevention [CDC] 2010). In NYC, MSM compose the largest proportion of new HIV/AIDS diagnoses (Torian et al. 2009); Black MSM have twice the number of new diagnoses as White MSM (New York City Department of Health and Mental Hygiene [NYCDOHMH] 2007). Taken together, these data suggest that, without a heightened community-level response aimed at reducing risk and vulnerability to HIV, the HIV epidemic will continue to rage among Black MSM. The need for community-level responses to prevent HIV/AIDS among Black MSM is noted in the *National HIV/AIDS Strategy* (White House 2010) and has been called for by researchers and policy-makers (Kegeles et al. 1996, Bing et al. 2008, Wilson and Moore 2009).

Methods

We conducted interviews and focus groups at churches in predominantly Black (i.e., African-American, Afro-Caribbean and/or African immigrant) neighbourhoods in NYC. Most of the churches included in the study engaged in HIV prevention or other HIV-related efforts on some level (e.g., sponsored information sessions on HIV, engaged in HIV testing efforts, participated in The Balm in Gilead's *National Week of Prayer for the Healing of AIDS*, etc.). Some of the churches had HIV/AIDS ministries, which actively sought to mobilise church members, parishioners and community members in response to the HIV/AIDS epidemic.

Sample

A number of strategies were used to recruit participants. The first author collaborated with a local HIV/AIDS community-based organisation that was working with Black churches to develop HIV/AIDS ministries. Members of our research team also approached leaders at churches they were familiar with. Other participants were recruited through referrals. The resulting convenience sample consisted of 81 women and men representing 6 Baptist churches, three African Methodist Episcopal (AME) churches, two Catholic churches, three inter/non-denominational churches and one Presbyterian church. The churches included in the study were located in neighbourhoods with large Black populations in four boroughs (the Bronx, Brooklyn, Manhattan and Queens) of NYC. The participating churches were concerned with mobilising in response to the local HIV/AIDS epidemic. A sample of this type enabled us to explore ideologies among churches with the potential to become active players in the fight against HIV among Black MSM. We conducted a total of 10 focus groups with parishioners and 10 interviews with pastors and other church leaders. All but one of the church leaders interviewed were men. The majority of the participants were Black.

Interview and focus group protocols

Semi-structured interviews and focus groups were primarily conducted in churches. Interviews and focus groups lasted 1–2 hours and were audio recorded with the written consent of the participants. Interview and focus group topics focused on churches'/worship traditions' values related to sexuality (condom use, unprotected sex and homosexuality in particular); health and illness; stigma; and HIV/AIDS (including church responses to HIV/AIDS). Probes were used to explore issues and salient points raised. Interviews with pastors provided information on churches' official stances and decision-making processes, as well as insight into pastors' internal conflicts. The individual interviews also allowed us to have more intimate and detailed conversations with church leaders than would have been afforded in a group environment. Focus groups consisted of approximately 5–7 church parishioners. Focus groups provided parishioners with opportunities to delve deeply into issues and to discuss and debate their church's values with their peers. The use of focus groups enabled us to gain a better understanding of dynamics within the churches, as well as of which topics were least and most controversial.

Analytic approach

All interviews and focus groups were transcribed by a professional transcription company. We employed a multistage, iterative process in analysing transcripts. The analysis was guided by the principles of Grounded Theory (Strauss and Corbin 1990), in which key themes and codes used to organise themes emerge out of the data and are not determined a priori. The process included several steps. The first step involved reviewing transcripts and memoing. Memos were then compared and discussed, and a working codebook was developed; codes were added and their definitions refined over a series of meetings. We then engaged in a process of systematically coding each interview and focus group transcript. In this article, we focus on the following codes: 'Acceptance', 'Church Response', 'Community Mobilisation', 'Discrimination', 'HIV/AIDS', 'Homosexuality', 'Homophobia', 'Religious Ideology', 'Sin' and 'Stigma'. These codes were used to identify and compare themes. Themes were integrated into a finding matrix, which was used as a framework for condensing findings and fulfilling the research goals.

Findings

We sought to explore the relationship between church ideologies – of sexuality, bodies and HIV/AIDS – and church mobilisation, or lack thereof, in response to the HIV crisis affecting Black MSM. In general, church responses to HIV focused on support of and prayer for those who are sick, HIV/AIDS and sex education (e.g., health fairs, workshops and pastoral counselling), and referrals to prevention and treatment services in the community. A few churches engaged in condom distribution, while others considered it to be outside the realm of church-sanctioned activities; however, many recognised the importance of condoms as an effective way to maintain sexual health. For example, a male member of a non-denominational church in Brooklyn noted, 'While abstinence is the ideal we are very realistic about who our membership is and who the people in the community we serve are so we don't provide condoms but we will connect them with resources where they can take care of themselves'. None of the churches reported specifically responding to the crisis among Black MSM, nor did any address the reality that men are having sex with men within the context of HIV mobilisation activities. Only one church reported holding an HIV testing and education workshop for LGBT youth of faith. Our analysis of interview and focus group data revealed the following prominent themes, which can help explain the lack of MSM-focused mobilisation efforts:

(1) 'Love the sinner, hate the sin' (LSHS) – The belief that homosexual behaviour can be distinguished and separated from homosexual identity.
(2) 'Don't ask, don't tell' – The belief that homosexual identities and behaviours should be kept private.
(3) 'Your body is a temple' – The belief that spiritual and physical health are interconnected.

We discuss these findings in terms of their implications for church mobilisation in response to HIV among Black MSM.

'Love the sinner, hate the sin': behaviour vs. identity

When parishioners and pastors were asked about homosexuality, a common response across denominations was that Christians should 'love the sinner' but 'hate the sin'. As one female member of an HIV Ministry at an AME church in Queens stated:

> But the thing is we might not condone [homosexuality], but everybody is a child of God. So God doesn't say, 'I'm not gonna love you because you are a certain way'. But God says that [homosexual] behaviour is an abomination. So know it for what it is. And then govern yourself from that. So you know we have these discussions all the time, cause I have plenty of gay friends.

The specific phrase 'love the sinner, hate the sin' was referred to by many of our focus group and interview participants. For example:

> You know, I have a number of people who I interact with and, you know, and they are homosexual and I love them. One of the things that I know is that God loves people, but he might not love the sin, and the reason that God, I believe, is opposed to it is because it doesn't reproduce, okay? So two men can't reproduce and two women can't reproduce and that was the reason that God created them.
> —Female pastor, non-denominational, Brooklyn

Other participants alluded to the LSHS ideology by distinguishing between 'lifestyle' and 'the individual'.

> In our practice, we believe in the way that Jesus taught, which was that everyone deserves love. Everyone needs love. Everyone needs service and ministry. And so, we do our best not to judge, but just to love all. I mean that, you know, the church is open to all of God's children. And anyone who is seeking God is a child of God. However, you know, our church does not believe in male-to-male marriage or female-to-female marriage. We don't try to dive into peoples' bedrooms. But on our exterior, you know, we – the fundamentals of our theology will not allow us to promote the lifestyle, even though we love the individual.
> —Male Elder, AME, Bronx

A male pastor of an AME church in Washington Heights stated:

> I am decidedly and intentionally heterosexual. I make no bones about that. I have no issues with that. And I think God's intention for humanity was that men and women would be together. I think that was God's intention. Now, having said that, we realize that that's not what's happening in our society. I am obligated to love you even if I don't like what you do...So, I have taken the approach of I preach family and I preach that God's intention and design for family was a man and a woman. I teach that. But I have a number of homosexual men and lesbian women who are members of our church. Because I tell them upfront, 'Look, I love you. I'm not judging you. But here is where I am with this'. Now, having said that, if you can sit under my teaching and my preaching, I will never bash you, never make you feel uncomfortable, never make fun of you, never do any of that. But if you can get with that, then we're all right.

The same pastor later reiterated his understanding that homosexuality is a lifestyle that he does not support but that this has not stopped him from nominating gay and lesbian individuals to leadership positions:

We've hosted here conferences and workshops, LGBT conferences and things. We've hosted them. Not that I'm supportive of the lifestyle. But one of the reasons that I host it is because the church needs to be educated...it's all about exposure and education, and knowing – being confident in who you are as a person and what you believe. And to the point where I have even nominated person who I knew were gay or homosexual – gay or lesbian – to leadership positions in our church.

A male pastor of a Baptist church in Manhattan made a similar distinction between the 'lifestyle' and 'the person', describing how he has stood up for homosexuals:

And for a lot of people, and for a lot of homosexuals that I've counselled and befriended, and are friends to this day, and I mentor some, and gladly. And have learned how to stand up for them and use faith to defend them to a degree. Not their lifestyle, but to defend the person and their choice.

Like the AME pastor, this Baptist pastor referred to individual homosexuals who he has displayed his acceptance of, in this case through counselling, friendship and mentorship. In contrast, a male pastor of a Baptist church in Brooklyn suggested that because homosexual behaviour and identity are distinct, the latter can be maintained while the former is abandoned:

Now, having said that, the question becomes, ultimately, for me, a matter of whether you're straight or gay, do we allow our sexuality to dominate our choices? . . . So, in our community, you can be gay and still be saved as it were. The issue is not orientation. The issue is action.

Don't ask, don't tell: private vs. public knowledge

Some participants did not focus on homosexuality or same-sex sexuality as sinful, per se. They more or less accepted that homosexual behaviour occurs, but suggested that same-sex sexuality was a private matter that individuals should not disclose and that the church is not prepared to discuss. Tied to this understanding was the belief that sexuality – specifically homosexuality – was a superficial or insignificant characteristic of the person; homosexuality was contrasted with more important, substantial characteristics that, according to participants' theology, make the person who he or she is. For example, a female parishioner at a Baptist church in Manhattan stated:

Pastor said what we've done with homosexuality is we've minimised that person to what they do in the bedroom and that's exactly what we've done. They're still working men, they're still working women. They're still – you know – they are in the community, they do everything we do and then we make them so small as to what they do behind a closed door and if they knew what we did behind closed doors then it would be one of those things.

Parishioners and pastors discussed the importance of maintaining a separation between the public selves and private lives of members and placed same-sex behaviour within the latter sphere. This ideology is best described as 'don't ask, don't tell' (DADT), as participants explicitly described it. A female parishioner from a Presbyterian church in Brooklyn stated, 'I think it's pretty much like now where we – it's [homosexuality is] not discussed . . . don't ask, don't tell . . . everyone can be just together, but it's not really like discussed 'cause I guess we're not really faced or confronted with the issue of homosexuality'. Members of a Presbyterian church in Brooklyn noted that they welcome homosexual persons into the congregation, as long as they worship as 'regular' (parishioner's quotes) parishioners:

> Female: I mean for a person who has an open gay lifestyle, it's not open basically in the congregation. For the most part, they come in. If they do wanna worship, they worship as regular folks, quote, unquote, for the most part but there's no kind of outward hostility...
> Moderator: But it sounds like there's still an open policy—and tell me, please, if I'm wrong—that if a person is gay or lesbian or bisexual that they can come to this church. Is that correct?
> Female: Absolutely.
> Female: And they do.
> Male: Yeah, I think that it's basically don't ask, don't tell.
> Male: Same as the military, right?
> Female: Right.
> Male: I don't know what would happen if someone walked in openly gay with a gay partner...as far as membership is, I'm not sure what would happen.

Parishioners from a Catholic church in the Bronx expressed similar sentiments. However, these parishioners critiqued their church's silence around homosexuality, citing the presence of homosexual people in the congregation and the need to be open about same-sex behaviours:

> Male: People that you don't expect that, you know they do, whatever they doing in their life. And like I said, I'm not here to judge you. Let's talk about prevention. That's the most important part. But again, we have to talk like, push it under the table. Not wide open in church. And different people, they have different kind of – how would I put it? Life.
> Male: Lifestyle.
> Male: Lifestyle. You know. So we should be talking about it.
> Female: And it's been going on for – ...
> Male: [In the church] we do not talk about it. At all. It's not even mentioned. You might know of someone or whatever, you know but it's not mentioned at the pulpit. It's not mentioned nowhere. And people know this. People in our church of that lifestyle. But it's not even mentioned. And it's a taboo ... They will not speak on homosexuality.

Ignoring homosexuality and same-sex sexual behaviour or deeming it unimportant – and requesting that homosexual persons do not disclose their sexual orientation and/ or behaviour – was viewed as an improvement over hatred or condemnation. For example, parishioners at a Baptist church in Manhattan described their attitude towards homosexuality as follows:

> Male: When you live a life that's consumed by love you don't think about these other surface things, like, it just doesn't mean anything because I'm so concerned about loving you I don't care about how you identify yourself.
> Female: What you do behind closed doors ...
> Female: Because ultimately that's what it is.
> Male: Well I'm more concerned and I think God's more concerned about hearts than our genitalia.

Male: I think that's one – I've heard that from a preacher in a pulpit and, like, that just makes so much sense, like, we focus so much on outward things and don't focus on one another's hearts.

However, a male, non-denominational pastor in Brooklyn took a more aggressive stance:

What you do in your bed in the privacy of your home is your business. But why are you now putting it out in my face? Okay. Why do I even have to know what you're doing? ... I can love you. I'm looking beyond the fault and I see the need. You need God. Cause you just don't get it. God is love. But look, God loves the homosexual, but he doesn't love the behaviour. God loves the thief, but he doesn't love the stealing. God loves the murderer, but he doesn't love the killing.

This pastor's position, which connects the DADT and LSHS ideologies, reflects the ideas of other participants we interviewed. His way of responding to same-sex behaviour hinders open dialogue around homosexuality and, more specifically, HIV/AIDS among Black MSM. Moreover, while the pastor makes it clear that he does not condemn homosexual men and women, he does request that they keep their identities and behaviours private, which makes community mobilisation around HIV among Black MSM a nonstarter.

'Your body is a temple': physical health and spiritual health

Participants described the body as a temple and emphasised the importance of taking care of one's body, as an act of honouring God, and maintaining consistency between body and soul. The 'your body is a temple' (YBIT) phrase is taken directly from the Bible,[1] and many participants spoke about 'honouring your temple, which is your body', and noted that 'the Bible encourages us to live a healthy lifestyle'. For example, one female parishioner at a Baptist church in Manhattan stated: 'Your body is your temple. So, you're supposed to be striving to do good things for your body because that's the way you show faith, and that's the way you're able to show respect and gratitude for your blessings, by being the best you can be'.

Many parishioners and pastors emphasised that they did not believe HIV/AIDS was a punishment for sin or that anyone deserved to be infected. However, they made connections between the body and spirit and had a self-described 'holistic' understanding of physical and spiritual health. The YBIT ideology was helpful in that it facilitated church mobilisation around health issues and risk reduction. However, it was also problematic in that it allowed for the conflation of physical risk (i.e., for poor health outcomes such as HIV) and spiritual risk/sin. Participants spoke in vague terms when describing body-spirit connections in relation to HIV risk and prevention. In line with the DADT ideology, they did not specifically speak of homosexual behaviours or unprotected sex; rather, they spoke of taking care of oneself and behaving in accordance with Christian expectations. As a male priest at a Catholic church in the Bronx noted, 'Illness is part of life. Probably if you live long enough something is gonna happen to you. But am I doing the proper thing? Am I taking care of my body? So is my body a temple of the Holy Spirit?'.

Some participants failed to make distinctions between risky behaviours (such as unprotected sex and needle sharing) and sinful/immoral behaviours (such as non-marital sex and drug use) – or differences in the consequences of these behaviours. These pastors and parishioners suggested that if a behaviour is sinful then it is also bad for your physical health. The negative views of same-sex behaviour that some participants held were buttressed by the fact that MSM experience high rates of HIV. For example, a pastor at a Baptist church in Queens suggested that harming oneself and sinning are inextricably tied:

> It's a missing of His mark completely. What He originally planned. Just total disregard...Do this. Don't do that. Cut and dry. Clear. But you do that when you're told not to do that...that's going to create things. Because if you do what you're supposed to do, other things won't happen. [If you don't] illness happens. You create [illness]...you'll affect the body. If you did what you were supposed to do, it shouldn't affect this, which would not cause illness.

The understanding of the strong link between body and soul helps to explain the connections that were drawn (and the distinctions that were overlooked) between sinful and physically risky behaviours. Although HIV was not presented as a direct punishment for sin, some participants suggested that those who had contracted HIV as a result of sinful behaviour were more deserving of the virus than those who had contracted it by other means. One leader of an AME church in the Bronx, in discussing causes of HIV, described his understanding of the difference between 'mercy' and 'justice', which he believed to apply differently to people who have contracted HIV in different ways:

> Our Christian faith teaches us that we are all sinners, who have been given the right to forgiveness, because of the grace and kindness of our benevolent God. Innocent people don't need mercy. Guilty people need mercy...we're all guilty of something...However, there are some people who deserve justice, because they are innocent to a certain extent in their particular circumstance. And they should not have to suffer as it pertains to their particular circumstance that they had no way of changing. For example, people who are starving and hungry in a world where we have plenty of food. Why should – that is unjust...Or someone who may have been in prison for a crime they did not commit. For a person, you know, a child who was born with HIV and AIDS, who had – whose behaviour had nothing to do with the reason why they're infected. You know, they don't [sic] need justice. Someone who used drugs for years and years and years, who was a prostitute for years and they contracted HIV, they don't need justice, they need mercy...The person who was born with it and had no – they don't need mercy, they need justice.

An HIV-positive man who was in the HIV Ministry at an AME church in Queens echoed this sentiment:

> Thank God I was raised the right way. I didn't do anything wrong. It's something that happened. I don't know why. I might have been living immorally meaning I might have had more than one girlfriend. But I wasn't a homosexual man. I didn't use IV drugs. So when you take those two immoral things out the way...

The YBIT ideology may represent a missed opportunity for HIV prevention and mobilisation for several of the churches in the study. The pervasive focus on body-spirit connection facilitated the understanding that a healthy soul/spirit breeds a healthy body and vice versa. This focus also reinforced the idea that an unhealthy soul/spirit breeds an unhealthy body and vice versa. The body-spirit connection was often used by pastors and parishioners as a way to promote (or discourage) certain lifestyles, as opposed to a way to reduce HIV risk and promote prevention. A few churches promoted the ideology in such a way that protecting one's body meant staying safe and healthy when engaging in behaviours that may be labelled sinful. At an AME church in Manhattan – perhaps the most actively engaged in HIV prevention activities among all of the churches we explored – parishioners spoke of using the body-spirit connection in the context of risk reduction:

> Female: We have to protect ourselves. The only way we protect ourselves is through a barrier mass, to have a barrier there. We do not condone the kids to have – you know, there's a free will of choice. Your body is the temple of God and if you go take – step out, cover yourself. . . .
> Male: You have to protect yourself because you love you and our pastor talks about loving and if a person loves you enough they'll go and get tested, but in the meantime, if you won't wanna do all that because we are flesh and we want to enjoy sex, here are some condoms. We have a variety of condoms for whatever needs you might have.

A leader at an AME church in the Bronx distinguished between the theology and the liberal practice of his and other churches:

> Interviewer: What does the church say about condoms?
> Interviewee: Our church does not have a specific theology around condoms. We do teach that sex was created for the confines of marriage. Sex outside of marriage is not God ordained. That is our fundamental doctrine. Our liberal practice says, don't catch HIV. If you find yourself in the situation where you are not going to be able to abstain, have enough good sense to put on a condom.
> Interviewer: And would that ever come out of the mouth of the pastor?
> Interviewee: Yes. It's come out the mouths of many pastors that I know ... we preach, first, don't have sex, then you won't have to worry about catching any disease. You won't have to worry about getting pregnant, when you don't want your baby and none of that. However, we understand our human desire is very – our sexual desire is one of the most powerful desires that we have, if not the most powerful desire, and can move us to do some stupid things. And, you know, one of them is to have sex in an irresponsible way. So, you know, make sure that you're, at the very least, responsible.

Though this leader suggests that his views and practices are shared by others church leaders, our findings suggest that many Black churches may struggle with this approach. Moreover, no church used the YBIT ideology as a way to promote condom use specifically among MSM; when employed as a prevention strategy, it was most often spoken of in the context of premarital sex.

The LSHS and DADT ideologies facilitated distinctions between homosexual identities and behaviours, while the YBIT belief facilitated the conflation of health risks and spiritual risks. Both impeded mobilisation focused on reducing HIV among Black MSM. However, as the previous two quotes suggest, it is feasible for many churches to struggle with the morality of certain sexual behaviours while still supporting and promoting health among congregants and community members who engage in those behaviours.

Conclusion

We uncovered three inter-related ideologies tied to sexuality and health in exploring responses to HIV among Black MSM among Black churches in NYC. As expected, parishioners' and pastors' opinions surrounding HIV/AIDS, sexuality in general, and homosexuality in particular were progressive in contrast to more fundamentalist churches' views (Miller 2007, Jeffries *et al.* 2008, Pitt 2010). These opinions allowed for acceptance of MSM despite condemnation of homosexual behaviours. However, because of the dualities and conflicts – between behaviours and identities, public knowledge and private actions, and health risks and sexual ones – embedded in these ideologies, effective HIV prevention efforts (i.e., involving condom use and harm reduction approaches) targeting Black MSM are difficult to mount.

The LSHS ideology, which repeatedly came up in focus groups and interviews, is not unique to Black churches in NYC; indeed it is promoted throughout Christian religious ideology (Jakobsen and Pellegrini 2004, Cheng 2010) and has been observed in other studies focusing on the church and homosexuality (Miller 2007, Barnes 2009). This ideology shuns sinful behaviour while focusing on loving and supporting the person who engages in it. A similar but distinct ideology – referred to as 'don't ask, don't tell' – was uncovered through our analysis. When respondents expressed their commitment to loving all people in spite of their 'external' flaws, mistakes and sins, they also suggested that homosexuality should be kept private (i.e., that people should not disclose their non-heterosexual orientation or behaviour). However, ignoring sexual orientation and/or deeming it unimportant poses a significant barrier to frank discussion about same-sex sexual behaviour. Research on the Black church has emphasised sexual silence as a key barrier to HIV prevention and sexual health promotion efforts (West 1993, Douglas 1999, Quimby and Friedman 2003, Hicks *et al.* 2005, Barnes 2009). Indeed, the barriers that many Black churches in our study faced in mounting MSM-focused prevention efforts did not stem from hatred of homosexuals or inability to accept and support MSM; rather, these barriers came from an inability to accept and talk about the sexual behaviours that occur between men and that are tied to HIV risk.

Dialogue around homosexuality and same-sex behaviours is necessary to reduce HIV risk among BMSM and stimulate mobilisation around HIV. McKenzie (2004) explored the relationship between dialogue and mobilisation within the context of Black churches' political activities. He suggested that dialogue and informal discussion produce 'action contexts', which he describes as 'situations that change the salience of collective action efforts by making them immediately and personally relevant to individuals' (p. 623). Dialogue and information sharing among parishioners – from giving testimony during service to chatting with other members in Sunday school – stimulates consciousness-raising and social action (McKenzie 2004, Hicks *et al.* 2005). The churches examined in this study have the potential to create action contexts through promoting dialogue around homosexuality. However, church endorsement of the LSHS and DADT ideologies must be critically examined as a probable barrier to effective community mobilisation.

While the LSHS and DADT ideologies represent barriers to community-level prevention, the YBIT ideology represents a missed opportunity for church-based efforts to prevent HIV among Black MSM. The common understanding that spiritual and physical health are inter-connected has promoted attention to health issues among church parishioners and leaders. The link between spiritual and physical health (i.e., the message of YBIT) can be used for HIV prevention/condom promotion, but can also serve to universally condemn same-sex behaviour. This ideology could be leveraged to promote self-care as an act of Christian devotion. However, the linking of physical risk and sin (spiritual risk) may serve as a barrier to HIV prevention and mobilisation activities (Malebranche 2003). By conflating risky behaviour and sinful behaviour, parishioners and leaders limit opportunities for harm reduction approaches to HIV prevention. A few churches held the viewpoint that morally questionable behaviours do not necessarily have to be physically unhealthy behaviours; this enabled them to employ a harm reduction focus to HIV prevention (e.g., condom distribution). However, several congregations failed to distinguish behaviours that negatively impact one's health from those that negatively impact one's spirit.

The pastors and parishioners that participated in this study shared the idea that taking care of health is a way of showing commitment to God. Using condoms and engaging in other risk reduction practices – though health-preserving actions – were not emphasised as ways of being committed to one's Christian faith. The 'body as temple' ideology could serve as a quintessential message of protection and harm reduction; however, for many of the churches in this study, it was an ideology used to reinforce views that denigrate homosexuality and same-sex behaviour, thereby undermining effective prevention.

There are three key limitations to this research that affect the interpretation of our findings and that should be highlighted. First, the findings reported here are not generalisable to all Black churches in the USA or in NYC. The size and nature of this sample, along with our analytic approach, prohibit us from drawing general conclusions about ideologies that facilitate or hinder effective responses to HIV in Black MSM among all NYC-based Black churches. Our sample enabled us to explore ideologies among churches with the potential to become active players in the fight against HIV among Black MSM. Thus, we were able to explore both potential barriers to and potential facilitators of mobilisation in response to HIV among Black MSM. Second, we did not attempt to collect data from gay, bisexual or other MSM parishioners or pastors. While these men were undoubtedly a part of the congregations we studied and the focus groups we conducted, our aim was not to focus on the individual perspectives of Black MSM in the church, but rather to describe institutional perspectives on Black MSM and the HIV crisis affecting them. There is a growing body of research that has focused on the former (e.g., Woodyard *et al.* 2000, Miller 2007, Jeffries *et al.* 2008, Pitt 2010) though very little work on the latter. Nonetheless, more work is needed to obtain views from Black MSM on the ways that Black churches can mobilise against HIV and engage in a dialogue around homosexuality. Finally, we did not explore differences in ideologies of churches of different denominations nor did we examine church responses to HIV by denomination. Our goal was to explore ideologies and church responses across denominations of Black churches. However, it is reasonable to assume that certain denominations could have more or less strict/lenient ideological stances, which could have differential impacts on mobilisation. These denominational differences should be explored in future studies.

In spite of the limitations of the research, this study makes valuable contributions to our understanding of the ideologies of Black churches and their impacts on

HIV/AIDS mobilisation. More specifically, the study provides insight into those church messages and doctrines that may hinder open dialogue and church mobilisation against HIV among Black MSM (i.e., LSHS and DADT), as well as those that may be used to facilitate mobilisation (i.e., YBIT). Black churches in NYC have a long history of rallying against problems affecting the community and can draw upon this history in mobilising to fight HIV among Black MSM. Ideologies that thwart conversation around homosexuality should be scrutinised and used to foster dialogue. Our findings specifically point to the YBIT ideology, as well as the LSHS and DADT ideologies (though perhaps not as directly), as a potential springboard for open dialogue about harm reduction in sexual encounters. Such dialogue might address questions including: How does LSHS work in practice? If DADT does not work for the US military, how well can it work for the church, and for individuals engaging in same-sex sexual relationships? And, if my body is a temple, should I not protect it all costs to celebrate God? The dialogues that come about from open discussion of these questions within congregations can have consciousness-raising effects that can lead to church-based action (McKenzie 2004). Indeed, Black churches have a particularly rich history of applying Christian ideology to the specific, present-day struggles of African-Americans. This is a moment in time for Black churches to consider the LSHS, DADT and YBIT ideologies in the context of the crisis of HIV among BMSM.

Acknowledgements

This research was supported by grant 3 R01HD050118-S1 (awarded to Richard G. Parker, Ph.D. by the Eunice Kennedy Shriver National Institute of Child Health and Human Development), a diversity supplement to the parent grant RO1-HD050118, which supported a research study entitled Religious Responses to HIV/AIDS in Brazil. This article was also supported by a Eugene Kennedy Shriver US National Institute of Child Health and Human Development administrative supplement to this parent grant (grant number 3 R01HD050118-05S1; Principal Investigator Richard G. Parker, Ph.D.), issued under the American Recovery and Reinvestment Act of 2009. The views expressed in this paper are solely those of the authors and not those of NICHD.

Note

1. The 'body is a temple' phrase comes from 1 Corinthians 6:19-20 (New International Version): 'Do you not know that *your body is a temple* of the Holy Spirit, who is in you, whom you have received from God? You are not your own; you were bought at a price. Therefore honour God with your body'.

References

Barnes, S.L., 2005. Black church culture and community action. *Social Forces*, 84 (2), 967–994.
Barnes, S.L., 2009. The Influence of Black church culture: how Black church leaders frame the HIV/AIDS discourse. *Journal of Inter-Religious Dialogue* [online], 2. Available from: http://irdialogue.org/journal/issue02/the-influence-of-black-church-culture-how-black-church-leaders-frame-the-hivaids-discourse-by-sandra-l-barnes/ [Accessed 25 May 2011].
Bing, E.G., Bingham, T., and Millett, G.A., 2008. Research needed to more effectively combat HIV among African-American men who have sex with men. *Journal of the National Medical Association*, 100 (1), 52–56.

Bunche, R.I., 1973. *The political status of the Negro in the age of FDR*. Chicago: University of Chicago Press.

Centers for Disease Control and Prevention (CDC), 2010. Prevalence and awareness of HIV infection among men who have sex with men: 21 cities, United States, 2008. *Morbidity and Mortality Weekly Report*, 59 (37), 1201–1207.

Cheng, P.S., 2010. "Love the sinner, hate the sin" and other modern-day heresies. *Huffington Post* [online], 6 April. Available from: http://www.huffingtonpost.com/rev-patrick-s-cheng-phd/love-the-sinner-hate-the_b_526355.html [Accessed 25 May 2011].

Davis, N., 2008. HIV/AIDS and the black church: a qualitative multiple-case study investigation. Paper presented at the annual United States Conference on AIDS, Ft. Lauderdale, FL.

Douglas, K.B., 1999. *Sexuality and the black church*. Maryknoll, NY: Orbis Books.

Fullilove, M.T. and Fullilove, R.E., 1999. Stigma as an obstacle to AIDS action. *The American Behavioral Scientist*, 42 (7), 1117–1129.

Griffith, D.M., Campbell, B., Allen, J.O., Robinson, K.J., and Stewart, S.K., 2010. Your blessed health: an HIV-prevention program bridging faith and public health communities. *Public Health Reports*, 125 (S1), 4–11.

Harris, F.C., 1999. *Something within: religion in African-American political activism*. Cary, NC: Oxford University Press.

Harris, A.C., 2009. Marginalization by the marginalized: race, homophobia, heterosexism, and "the problem of the 21st century". *Journal of Gay & Lesbian Social Services*, 21 (4), 430–448.

Hicks, K.E., Allen, J.A., and Wright, E.M., 2005. Building holistic HIV/AIDS responses in African American urban faith communities. *Family & Community Health*, 28 (2), 184–205.

Jakobsen, J.R. and Pellegrini, A., 2004. *Love the sin: sexual regulation and the limits of religious tolerance*. Boston: Beacon Press.

Jeffries, W.L., Dodge, B., and Sandfort, T.G.M., 2008. Religion and spirituality among bisexual Black men in the USA. Culture. *Health & Sexuality*, 10 (5), 463–477.

Kegeles, S.M., Hays, R.B., and Coates, T.J., 1996. The Mpowerment Project: a community-level HIV prevention intervention for young gay men. *American Journal of Public Health*, 86 (8), 1129–1136.

Lincoln, C.E. and Mamiya, L.H., 1990. *Black church in the African-American experience*. Durham: Duke University Press.

Madison, A.-M. and McGadney, B.F., 2000. Collaboration of churches and service providers: meeting the needs of older African Americans. *Journal of Religious Gerontology*, 11 (1), 23–37.

Malebranche, D.K., 2003. Black men who have sex with men and the HIV epidemic: next steps for public health. *American Journal of Public Health*, 93 (6), 862–865.

McClerking, H.K. and McDaniel, E.L., 2005. Belonging and doing: political churches and black political participation. *Political Psychology*, 26 (5), 721–734.

McKenzie, B.D., 2004. Religious social networks, indirect mobilization, and African-American political participation. *Political Research Quarterly*, 57 (4), 621–632.

Miller, R.L., Jr, 2007. Legacy denied: African American gay men, AIDS, and the black church. *Social Work and Society*, 25 (1), 51–61.

Nelson, M., 2005. Let the choir say "amen": the impact of intragroup perceptions on African Americans with HIV/AIDS. *In*: D.A. Harley and J.M. Dillard, eds. *Contemporary mental health issues among African Americans*. Alexandria, VA: American Counseling Association, 107–118.

New York City Department of Health and Mental Hygiene (NYDOHMH), 2007. *New HIV diagnoses rising in New York City among young men who have sex with men: young Blacks and Hispanics hit hardest* [online]. Available from: http://www.nyc.gov/html/doh/html/pr2007/pr079-07.shtml [Accessed 25 May 2011].

O'Connor, T., Ryan, P., and Parikh, C., 1998. A model program for churches and ex-offender reintegration. *Journal of Offender Rehabilitation*, 28 (1&2), 107–126.

Pattillo-McCoy, M., 1998. Church culture as a strategy of action in the Black community. *American Sociological Review*, 63 (6), 767–784.

Pew Forum on Religion & Public Life, 2008. *U.S. religious landscape survey.* Washington, DC: Pew Research Center.

Pitt, R.N., 2010. "Killing the Messenger": religious Black gay men's neutralization of anti-gay religious messages. *Journal for the Scientific Study of Religion,* 49 (1), 56–72.

Quimby, E. and Friedman, S.R., 2003. Dynamics of Black mobilization against HIV/AIDS in New York City. *In*: P. Conrad and V. Leiter, eds. *Health and health care as social problems.* Lanham, MD: Rowman and Littlefield, 145–159.

Shapiro, L.D., Thompson, D., and Calhoun, E., 2006. Sustaining a safety net breast and cervical cancer detection program. *Journal of Health Care for the Poor and Underserved,* 17 (2), 20–30.

Spencer, J.M., 1996. The black church and the Harlem Renaissance. *African American Review,* 30 (3), 452–460.

Strauss, A. and Corbin, J., 1990. *Basics of qualitative research: grounded theory procedures and techniques.* Newbury Park, CA: Sage Publications.

Taylor, R., Mattis, J., and Chatters, L., 1999. Subjective religiosity among African Americans: a synthesis of findings from five national samples. *Journal of Black Psychology,* 25 (4), 524–543.

Torian, L.V., Forgione, L.A., Eavey, J., Kent, S., and Bennani, Y., 2009. HIV incidence in New York City in 2006. Poster presented at the 16th Conference on Retroviruses and Opportunistic Infections, Montreal, Canada.

United States Department of Health and Human Services (DHHS), 2010. *Presidential Advisory Council on HIV/AIDS-Secretary Sebelius announces members of the Presidential Advisory Council on HIV/AIDS* [online]. Available from: http://www.whitehouse.gov/administration/eop/onap/pacha [Accessed 25 May 2011].

West, C., 1993. Black culture and postmodernism. *In*: L. Hutcheon and J. Natoli, eds. *A postmodern reader.* Albany: State University of New York Press, 390–397.

White House Office of National AIDS Policy, 2010. *National HIV/AID strategy for the United States* [online]. Washington, DC. Available from: http://www.whitehouse.gov/sites/default/files/uploads/NHAS.pdf [Accessed 3 May 2010].

Wilson, P.A. and Moore, T.E., 2009. Public health responses to the HIV epidemic among Black men who have sex with men: a qualitative study of US health departments and communities. *American Journal of Public Health,* 99 (6), 1013–1022.

Woodyard, J.L., Peterson, J.L., and Stokes, J.P., 2000. "Let us go into the house of the Lord": participation in African American churches among young African American men who have sex with men. *Journal of Pastoral Care,* 54 (4), 451–460.

Vulnerable salvation: Evangelical Protestant leaders and institutions, drug use and HIV and AIDS in the urban periphery of Rio de Janeiro

Jonathan Garcia[a], Miguel Muñoz-Laboy[b] and Richard Parker[b]

[a]Center for Interdisciplinary Research on AIDS, Yale School of Public Health, Yale University, New Haven, CT, USA; [b]Department of Sociomedical Sciences, Mailman School of Public Health, Columbia University, New York, NY, USA

This analysis focuses on the evangelical Protestant responses to drug use and HIV prevention, treatment and care in the urban periphery of Rio de Janeiro. We question how religious institutions, and the positions of pastors, create or reduce various elements of societal illness and vulnerability. We aim to show that the views of pastors may symbolise a form of social regulation that may have a meaningful social impact on drug use and HIV and AIDS. The interviews of 23 evangelical religious leaders were collected. Two case studies of evangelical drug rehabilitation centres (DRC) are derived from five qualitative interviews. Evangelical DRC generally reflects pastors' discourses of reintegration into social networks including marriage, family and employment. We found important differences in the discourses and practices in private versus state-funded rehabilitation centres that may reveal ways social and programmatic vulnerabilities may affect the efficacy of public health interventions.

Introduction

The proliferation of evangelical, especially Pentecostal, religions has been a world-wide phenomenon (Hunt 2000).[1] Globalising religious groups have not only formed transnational linkages, but they have also focused on establishing deep roots on the local level with distinct cultural interpretations (Hunt 2000). The health disparities in developing countries have presented challenges to the 'wealth and health' gospel. In low- and middle-income countries and regions, a number of scholars have documented the importance of evangelical religious groups in strategising to mitigate problems linked with HIV and drug use, which have affected populations that are socio-economically and culturally marginalised (Todd et al. 2007, Hansen 2004).

Religious leaders and institutions could mould perceptions about HIV-related vulnerabilities (Smith 2004, Adogame, 2007, Eriksson et al. 2010) and drug use (Todd et al. 2007, Deng et al. 2007, Sanchez and Nappo 2008). Religious institutions, especially the rapidly proliferating evangelical groups, have high levels of community influence in impoverished and culturally marginalised communities in Rio de Janeiro that are considered to be the most vulnerable to HIV (Garcia et al. 2009). They may play an integral role in improving health indicators and social cohesion. Religions offer options for participation in the social world (Chesnut 2003). Religious organisations have stepped in to solve such 'pathogens of poverty' (Chesnut 1997). In fact the 'pathogens of poverty' can be termed the 'pathogens of inequality' if we consider the role of racism, gender inequality, unemployment, discrimination based on sexual orientation, etc., in these areas. The role of evangelical religious institutions has been interpreted as a response to the societal illness and structural violence suffered by poor and marginalised women and men (Burdick 1993, Chesnut 2003).

Drug use and HIV have been considered societal illnesses. In Brazil, a total of 22.7% reported cases of AIDS were due to intravenous drug use in 1997, decreasing to 7.2% by 2008 (Brazilian Ministry of Health 2008). In a multisite epidemiological study conducted in 10 Brazilian cities (Rio de Janeiro, Manaus, Recife, Salvador, Belo Horizonte, Santos, Curitíba, Itajaí, Campo Grande and Brasília), Bastos (2009) found that the prevalence among drug users was 5.9%, much higher than the national prevalence of 0.7% in the general population. The decrease in cocaine injection has given way to a rise in the use of crack, which is associated with higher levels of sexual risk behaviours (Pechansky *et al.* 2006, Azevedo *et al.* 2007). Drug use, ranging from crack (Azevedo *et al.* 2007), to marijuana and alcohol, is still a major concern for curbing the AIDS epidemic in Brazil (Garcia and Siqueira 2005, Pechansky *et al.* 2006). The synergistic epidemic of drug use and HIV is exacerbated by other societal problems, primarily due to *vulnerabilities* related to poverty, race and sexuality, which tear at the social fabric. In the last decade, the Ministry of Health and the National Secretariat against Drugs (SENAD) has proposed the involvement and regulation of religious groups involved in drug rehabilitation (Garcia and Siqueira 2005).

The concept of vulnerability brings together individual, social and programmatic elements of the processes such as the policy negotiation, the production of knowledge and the invention of technologies for sociocultural and structural health interventions (Ayres 1996, Paim and Filho 1998, Ayres *et al.* 2003, Ayres *et al.* 2006). The social vulnerability framework has been used mostly in HIV research to counterbalance behavioural approaches, which are said to attribute shame and blame to individuals that engage in risky behaviours (Delor and Hubert 2000). Social ties can reinforce a variety of norms and behaviours, such as the conceptualisations of health and illness (Kawachi and Berkman 2000). Vulnerability can denote a *process* where personal agency is shaped and limited by a dominant culture.

Programmatic vulnerability relates to the processes of governance and intervention that shape individual agency and social structures. The WHO defined programmatic vulnerability as having three fundamental components, 'information and education, health and social services, and non-discrimination' (Mann and Tarantola 1996, p. 441). Some argue that in places where the state is weak, informal institutions act as substitutes in the provision of social goods (Isham *et al.* 2002). These social and political stakeholders affect the 'availability and accessibility of key programme elements, the quality and content of each element, and the process through which the elements are designed, implemented, and evaluated' (Mann and Tarantola 1996, p. 442). Both structures (programmes) and individuals (service recipients) can be affected by programmatic vulnerability.

Where the health system and the state have failed to reach large portions of the population, evangelical religious institutions and leaders have played a significant role in providing drug-related health services in Brazil (Sanchez and Nappo 2008). This paper uses the concepts of social and programmatic vulnerability to analyse the ways evangelical communities and institutions can address issues related to drug use and HIV. Whereas attempting to decrease drug and alcohol use may reduce vulnerability, claims that physical illness can be cured through spiritual rituals add a level of concern for HIV- and AIDS-related community interventions. First, the discourses of evangelical religious leaders are presented to uncover some elements of how religious leaders may frame vulnerabilities related to drug use and HIV. Then, two case studies of evangelical rehabilitation centres present an institutional perspective, contrasting ideological and pragmatic approaches that may depend on institutional relationships with the state.

Methods

Research site and social context

This study was conducted in the *Baixada Fluminense,* the urban periphery of Rio de Janeiro, between December 2006 and March 2009 as part of a larger study on the religious responses to HIV and AIDS in Brazil.[2] The living conditions of the *Baixada Fluminense* are historically marked by high levels of poverty, attributed in part to geographic confinement and segregation due to urbanisation (CIDE 2005, Garcia *et al.* 2009). According to Chesnut (1997), a 'huge labor surplus, even in the context of economic growth, ensures that salaries will not rise' (p. 15). Much of this population survives in precarious housing conditions and poorly functioning sanitation (CIDE 2005).

Moreover, the relationship between poor health and life expectancy in urban poor Rio de Janeiro and areas with the highest proportion of residents of poor communities and shantytowns suggests an environmental element of social disorganisation, emphasising the importance of social cohesion as a resource (Szwarcwald *et al.* 2000). The more comprehensive analyses of health disparities are not simply measured by 'hospital health' but by 'environments in which people live' showing that 'the residential environment cannot be simply considered as a compositional effect but rather as a contextual effect' (Szwarcwald *et al.* 2000, p. 534).

The absence of the state creates an ideal situation for the 'parallel governance' by drug traffickers. According to Soares (1996), the parallel power of drug trafficking leads to a lack of transparency and to corruption in the penal system – leaving 90% of criminal cases open without a search for the identity of the assassins. The *Baixada Fluminense* is the area in metropolitan Rio with some of the highest rates of violence, in comparison to other cities in Brazil (Human Rights Watch 2009). In fact, in these municipalities there is less than one police officer for 1000 people (CIDE 2005). Many deaths are caused by extermination by the police – officially justified as armed confrontations with local militia forces (Cano 1999). According to Marcelo Freixo, from the Centre for Global Justice, what is necessary is 'security as a citizen', including 'rights to housing, to employment, to health, [and] to education', which Freixo claims do not truly exist in metropolitan Rio de Janeiro (Martins 2004, Nadanvosky *et al.* 2009).

Sample selection and recruitment

We began sampling based on the Brazilian Interdisciplinary AIDS Association's (ABIA) network of AIDS-related NGOs. From this sample we identified two evangelical AIDS-related faith-based organisations (FBOs). We recruited six religious leaders from these two NGOs. From these two FBOs, we were referred to drug rehabilitation centres (DRC) run by evangelical pastors. We recruited five religious leaders from these centres. We continued our snowball sampling approach to expand our network of recruitment by asking the religious leaders who had agreed to participate in the study to indicate other leaders. Using this sampling technique, we recruited another 12 religious leaders from evangelical communities. Another 11 religious leaders were recruited through other evangelical FBOs and weak ties to ABIA. Our total sample included 23 evangelical religious leaders as shown in Figure 1. Generally, the trend shows that there are clusters of recruitment centred on the involvement of FBOs. These organisations were inter-denominational evangelical, but Pentecostals tended to recruit other Pentecostals. Both DRCs were associated with Pentecostal FBO_1 and FBO_2, and the state-funded DRC_2 tended to be located in a denser network than DRC_1.

The limitations of this study include the fact that only religious leaders were interviewed. Future studies should integrate an analysis of drug users with those of leaders. Interviewing drug users and people with HIV and AIDS brings out important elements of individual risk, but our attempt was to focus on the

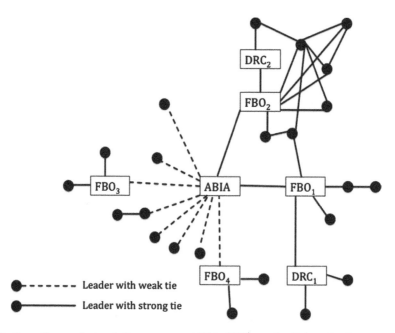

Figure 1. Sampling and associations among ABIA, FBOs and religious leaders.
Note: DRC, Drug Rehabilitation Centre; FBO, Faith-based Organization; ABIA, Brazilian Interdisciplinary AIDS Association.

institutions (and leaders as proxies for institutional codes) in order to capture social and programmatic dimensions of vulnerability. Although the case studies cannot be generalised to represent all DRCs, this approach points to essential factors influenced by organisational structures, funding and ideology.

Interviewing process and key questions

Qualitative interviews were conducted with evangelical pastors within the context of understanding their individual and institutional responses to AIDS, which included a component about drug use and HIV. The project's interview guide included open-ended and semi-structured questions. A research assistant with a background in HIV and social work conducted the interviews. Her knowledge of the religious field was crucial in order to form rapport with study participants, especially when asking sensitive questions regarding sexuality and drug use in their communities.

The first set of questions was regarding the individual religious leaders' perceptions and responses to the AIDS epidemic. Religious leaders were asked questions on (1) demographic data (age, marital status and monthly earnings); (2) questions about their religious communities (size, social work, gender and social problems); (3) their views on issues related to HIV and AIDS (including a history of their encounter with the epidemic, as well as their views on prevention, treatment and care for HIV and AIDS); and (4) questions on sexual and reproductive health (views on homosexuality, abortion, teenage pregnancy, fidelity and marriage).

The second set of questions was directed towards understanding the institutional responses of the religious group or FBO led by the religious leader. Institutional questions were used to construct case studies. These included (1) a historical trajectory of the institution including its funding and structure; (2) activities, related or unrelated to AIDS; (3) description of persons that use the services of the institution; (4) issues related to ideologies and the mission of the institution; (5) issues focused on the intersection between drug use and HIV risk (harm reduction, rehabilitation, abstinence and drug trafficking in their communities); and (6) articulation with civil society and the state.

Data analysis

Data were managed and kept securely at ABIA. The data were analysed using grounded theory (Glaser and Strauss 1967) through a selective coding technique. The authors open coded and verified observations using a qualitative codebook that was constructed manually. Then a spreadsheet in Microsoft Excel was used to compute data for all religious leaders. Key themes that were repeated in interviews were considered to have greater validity, and these were chosen for analysis in this article. Answers to open-ended or semi-structured questions related to drug use as it intersects with HIV vulnerabilities were of particular importance for this analysis. This intersection was the basis for selective coding into categories related to social vulnerabilities and programmatic vulnerabilities. Using discourse analysis, we aimed to contextualise the narratives of the religious leaders.

Results

Discourses of pastors

Drug trafficking urban poor Rio sets the backdrop for the involvement of evangelical churches on HIV. Through the decades, pastors in the *Baixada* have witnessed how youth are susceptible to working in the drug economy because 'even for those who do have the option of going to school and work, drug trafficking is a great subsidy that will get them money quickly', explained the coordinator of an evangelical AIDS NGO. This data reverts back to the expectations that poor neighbourhoods in geographically marginalised regions suffer from particular vulnerabilities.

> We know it should not be practiced, our society should seriously invest in combating drug trafficking and violence, but I am in favour of dialogue with these [drug gang] groups. I am also in favour of justice. But what is missing really is figuring out why it is all happening in poor communities on hillsides. (Presbyterian pastor for 11 years, congregation with 100 members)

We observed that the coexistence of religious institutions within drug-ruled communities is characterised by negotiation ('dialogue') in observation of territorialism. Religious organisations may need to support (or not contradict) drug trafficking governance in order to survive, although they are 'in favour of justice'. The negotiation necessary to work (or to conduct research) in poor areas with limited access to formal health care services is complicated and can be controlled by the legitimacy of religious organisations. These complex relations within civil society in places where there is an absence of the state create programmatic vulnerabilities that may be addressed through local community institutions, such as churches.

From the discourses of pastors, we found that drug use and the rehabilitation from addiction were key elements of evangelical cures for social problems, which could be interpreted as an attempt to cure vulnerability. Drug use was universally attributed to the manifestation of evil and in some cases demonic possession. All pastors used religious ideological discourses to regulate (or 'dominate' as argued by Bourdieu 1979) social interaction, at the same time that these discourses are strategic tools for welcoming those afflicted by the pathogens of inequality into the religion. While all churches welcomed drug users, there are elements of stigmatisation involved in the social processes of religious indoctrination.

> People who are dependent on drugs sometimes seek help . . . . So the Bible is rule that turns to practice. These [drug users] are immoral. It is our desire to rehabilitate them from the vice to spirituality. (Pentecostal pastor for 7 years, congregation with 400 members)

The ways of addressing vulnerability are not limited to adherence to the Scriptures, but they depend on the social interactions that occur in churches and on the effect that the family may have in providing social support. In this vein, another pastor makes a link between several social areas in which his church's *programmes* interact with its surrounding community, alluding to alcoholism, marriage and HIV.

> Our church's structure has programs for alcoholics, for marriage . . . because of poverty. [Our work] is called the Ministry of Family, of couples; we act in this area. And, working

with HIV, we could recuperate the community. (Baptist pastor for 4 years, congregation with 260 members)

Churches have programmes directed towards increasing social cohesion according to their ideologies. The greatest emphasis was on reincorporation into society, especially into the family and into work. One pastor emphasises the importance of the incorporation into the family and home for leading a healthy life.

> It is important that he enter into the path of a normal life, transformed. I have witnessed it. The family who thought there was no other way, and today is in the church in the path of the Lord, and I praise God for that. Now my worry is with their families. Why? The family always saw the things that they did wrong, the crimes they committed. We preach the Gospel and that the Lord Jesus Christ will help the person recuperate and return home. (Presbyterian pastor for 6 years, congregation with 140 members)

Table 1 summarises our findings based on selective coding, which map out how community formation and views of pastors regarding drug use and HIV may affect vulnerabilities. The table also shows solutions proposed for these problems that emerged most commonly in the interview narratives.

On another level, all pastors except for one thought abstinence and rehabilitation (not harm reduction) were the only ways to cure addiction and reincorporate people into society. The following pastor had to negotiate her actions and her discourses.

> My prevention is a bit radical, but it does not treat society as if it had no knowledge. I am in favour of the government in syringe exchange because there is a greater risk in injection drug users. I am in favour of government subsidies that do not view this as risk .... If I went on the pulpit of my church and preached that, they would say I was not a pastor .... In truth, I live a paradox. I live a constant war because I preach socialization and rehabilitation. (Ministry of Jesus, Pentecostal pastor for 8 years, congregation with 1300 members, leader at faith-based organization leader for AIDS services)

The pastor acts differently behind the pulpit than she does at her faith-based organisation. Her views at the pulpit may increase social vulnerability. Her work at the FBO may be considered an intervention that decreases programmatic vulnerability by providing services in marginalised populations that are hard to reach by

Table 1. Tiers of vulnerability and evangelical approaches to societal illness.

Vulnerability	Societal illness	Approaches/solutions
Individual	Overindulgence Libertinism Youth	Abstinence Spirituality/religious cures Psycho-spiritual treatment
Social	Disintegration of values Straying from community	Marriage Integration into family Employment
Programmatic	Lack of information Absence of state Drug economy	Church activities FBO participation Drug rehabilitation centre

the state. While this pastor shows openness to curbing transmission through injection drug use, there is still some lack of knowledge related to the risks of HIV infection associated with other drugs, such as crack cocaine.

Case study results

There may be a positive effect and reduction of social vulnerability through social integration. The idea of spiritual cures for social ills (including drug use and HIV) and the rejection of condoms by pastors may increase vulnerability within rehabilitation communities. The question remains of how these private or state-funded initiatives can affect programmatic vulnerability if we consider the state's outsourcing of social services to civil society organisations. The contrast between one centre that is funded privately by the community and another that is state-funded provides important insights about vulnerabilities addressed by contrasting institutional types and their approaches.

Case 1: Community and privately funded rehabilitation centre

The work with the spiritual and physical rehabilitation of men was inspired by a preacher who carried out a more 'institutionalised' version of the interviewee's first project. The pastor we interviewed organised and founded a halfway house, which received extremely negative responses from his neighbours. They created a legal petition to expel him from the community because he lived with vagabonds. He was surprised with the community's reaction considering that 'most of them were evangelical', and had to pause his work until he moved to another municipality. There he constructed – this time with donations and volunteer manual labour from neighbours – his first shelter, which also developed with contributions from evangelical churches in its environs.

After two decades, the centre offers services such as housing, feeding and establishing personal hygiene for male drug users. The facility now houses 41 men. The funding comes from the evangelical churches, community donations and assistance from some private companies ('with hearts moved by God'). There is no funding from the state, which 'makes the work difficult but God keeps them from scarcity', according to the pastor. The funding structure, as well as the mission of the institution determines the way the institution is organised, allowing for a small salaried staff of six social workers. The coordinator of the group acts as 'disciplinary figure' to the interned.

During the period of recuperation, which lasts approximately 9 months, there is a continued effort to reincorporate the person into his own family, if he has one. He becomes a volunteer at the institution if no family network is found. Those who do not wish to participate in religious activities are expelled from the facility, indicating the strong emphasis on indoctrination – for 'they must obey the leaders; if they do not obey the leaders it is not possible to carry out the work of recuperation', claims the pastor. The discipline given through work is part of the process of reintegration into society and communities, and it includes providing basic rights for these men through legal registration, identity cards, the equivalent social security number and a work card.

Moreover, the 'majority of the men interned at this facility are HIV positive, but they are not open about it', according to the pastor. In most cases only the staff knows, while in other cases it is visible that they are living with AIDS but do not want to admit it. One problem that created programmatic vulnerability was the delay in the HIV testing process because of the inefficiency of the health care system. It took 6 months to attain HIV test results. Due to the lack of facilities in the *Baixada Fluminense*, this process is slower, displaying a great concern for programmatic vulnerability. The fact that there are few facilities also creates greater external and auto-stigma because people are afraid of being seen by others in their own communities.

The pastor talked about an HIV positive man at the institution that had been involved in drug trafficking. The man believed that 'he did not have to take medications, but God would cure him'. And 'when his viral load was undetectable, and he recuperated from drug use, it was a miracle'. The pastor 'respects' when the HIV positive person 'truly believes and places his faith on spiritual cure'.

> We understand from the Bible that he who believes receives victory in Christ. We had an HIV positive man who needed treatment; God would cure him. In the Bible there is a text in which a blind man screamed 'Jesus have mercy on me', and in this plea, he wanted Jesus to cure him. When Jesus came closer to him, he asked, 'what is it you want? I will do it'. If the blind man asked to see, it is because he believed, so Jesus automatically cured him. So that happens today when the person confides, believes entirely that God can cure him. This was the case of this young man. Eventually, when he wanted to get married, he no longer needed to go to the doctor for treatment. (Pentecostal pastor and missionary, 20 years of service)

The organisation works with 'physical, moral and spiritual recuperation' and not with harm reduction, according to 'the work of God as written in the Bible'. The pastor believes that the way to prevent transmission of HIV is through what he calls the 'pact'. In what seems to be a contract, God stipulates, first, that abstinence should be practiced before marriage, and, second, that fidelity during marriage will protect the man and the woman from such diseases. Condoms are for those who break this pact, immediately attributing sin to their use.

Case 2: *State-funded rehabilitation centre*

This institution began over two decades ago as a drug rehabilitation community linked directly with an evangelical church. After the pastor founded the community, it was soon established as a state-funded clinic for drug dependency, with support from evangelical politicians. The pastor interviewed asserts the reason that this community was chosen for public funding was because 'the community has *know-how* in dealing with chemical dependence'. The structure of this entity and its areas of action are all related to treating facets of drug abstinence and rehabilitation. The NGO is directly related to a church in leadership and networks. The president is a pastor, and his wife and daughter are co-directors of the facility. All of the staff of the NGO belong to evangelical churches.

The organisation has approximately 90 workers, including doctors, psychiatrists, psychologists, social workers and nurses, among others, to provide 'bio-psycho-social' attendance. There are 190 persons receiving services, 170 men and 20 women.

In the interview, the pastor suggests that gender disparities may be due to the fact that men have 'tended to not adhere to treatment as well as women', and that the involvement of men in drug trafficking draws men closer to drug use. He offers an alternative explanation: 'the religiosity of women and adherence to belief systems that pronounce a cure is different than that of men', arguably making women less vulnerable.

> Not staying merely on the spiritual issues, we offer a fusion of the biotechnical and the spiritual, psychological. Before, the most [frequently] used drug was marijuana, it was the most offensive, but today it is cocaine and actually crack, a drug that destroys the capacity of thinking in the human. The NGO needed to be dynamic with such changes, not just focusing on the spiritual, providing incentives for the person to study psychology.... This is why we consider the technical and the spiritual, so that we can meet peoples' needs; it's not just a question of prayer. You need the point of view of medicine, and the social also. There should be a bio-psycho-social and spiritual approach. This wider view of the behaviour of the individual has been occurring since the foundation of the organization. (Coordinator of NGO)

In order to enter the facility, financed by the state, the subject goes through a triage with medical professionals that evaluate the condition of the drug user. Activities include: cleaning, individual consultation/treatment, talks, group meetings, 12-step groups and leisurely activities. Religious services are central but optional to avoid breaking the separation between church and state. As the pastor explains:

> We have, Wednesday at fourteen hours, Sundays from ten to eleven in the morning, but service is not an obligation, it's optional. It's important because it is a government project, which calls itself laical (laughs); you have respect. (Coordinator of NGO)

The organisation had some lectures on HIV and AIDS. The main topics of conversation were: (1) marriage and coping with AIDS, (2) employment and AIDS-related discrimination and (3) how to maintain social bonds when infected with HIV. The NGO does not work with HIV prevention through the distribution or promotion of condom use. When the pastor was asked whether the NGO supported condom use, there was a prolonged silence, and then he responded:

> It's not that the rehabilitation centre is in favour of the condom, but it's a double-edged sword. The NGO is in favour of sex as it was written in the Bible, of fidelity, after marriage. (Coordinator of NGO)

However, in this institution, AIDS is not seen as a punishment from God. Instead:

> Today this church is trying more and more to act without prejudice, through *information*. The church cannot stay restricted to the question of religion, as Jesus had a broader understanding of the human being, of human necessities. So for Him the leper did not shock him, [nor did] a prostitute. He gave them value, cured, and gave them words of hope and incentives. And today the church needs that – not to point at people. (Coordinator of NGO)

The ideas of access to information and linkages to other health services address important aspects of programmatic vulnerabilities encountered by institutions that treat drug users. The state could be passing-off responsibility for public drug rehabilitation to this centre because of its 'know-how', but the clear social norms against condom use create higher levels of vulnerability.

In comparing both case studies, there seems to be a stronger focus on spiritual cures in the privately funded centre, although the state-funded centre also supports spiritual cures for drug use and HIV if the person chooses to be saved (Table 2). In both cases there is strong emphasis on religious participation, an entirely evangelical staff and the possibility of spiritual cures. The state-funded institution integrates a 'bio-psycho-spiritual' approach to treatment through methods such as 12-step programmes, which comparatively lower vulnerabilities related to alienation. The scale of the state-funded centre is greater (41 members in case one versus 190 members in case two). There is also a difference in target populations. In the privately funded first case, only men are served, mostly homeless, while in case two 10.5% of those served are women. The emphasis on abstinence and marriage, as well as the symbolic prohibition of condoms creates a set of vulnerabilities. By comparing these two cases, it seems that state funding provides staff and infrastructure, as well as stricter guidelines, which make treatment closer to a biomedical model. Overall, we can say that state funding decreases programmatic vulnerability, but is it the duty of the state to provide these services directly or should these services be outsourced to religious groups?

Discussion and conclusions

This paper argued that values reinforced by social integration and inculcated religious ideology might be both barriers and facilitators to the pursuit of better health practices, particularly in addressing drug use and HIV. The frameworks of social and programmatic vulnerabilities developed early in the epidemic by Mann and Tarantola (1996) are employed to understand the quality of these health services, as they are mediated by discursive and programmatic intervention.

The framework of 'vulnerability' has been used frequently in HIV and AIDS research, but it has seldom been applied to drug use (Ayres *et al.* 2003). The paper offers an argument that religious institutions have a greater opening in places where the state has limited access to health, as was also indicated by studies such as Sanchez and Nappo (2008). This was true in poor, geographically marginalised

Table 2. Comparison of drug rehabilitation centres, according to sources of funding.

	Community and private funding	State funding
Composition	41 Men	170 Men and 20 women
Highest target population	Homeless men	Youth
Religious association	One evangelical church	Interdenominational evangelical churches
Methods for HIV prevention	Abstinence and fidelity in marriage, not condoms	Abstinence and fidelity in marriage, preferably not condoms
Treatment and care for drug use and AIDS	Spiritual cures, rehabilitation, social integration	Spiritual cures, rehabilitation, social integration, biomedical and psychological treatment

communities in the peri-urban Rio de Janeiro, where drug cartels have power to negotiate the actions of local institutions. The interactions and legitimacy of religious institutions may mitigate violence in the governance of these communities.

We first looked at the evangelical communities through the discourses of the evangelical pastors. We highlighted the importance of religious institutions in these communities and implications of vulnerabilities associated with the 'pathogens of poverty' (Chesnut 1997) or rather the pathogens of inequality. We found that in the evangelical discourses regarding drug use and HIV there may be increased social and programmatic vulnerability by advocating spiritual cures and not accepting harm reduction in some cases. Religious institutions and leaders reinforce community values and morals. These may be ideologically and symbolic domination (Bourdieu 1979) driven by scriptures, the social agendas of religious leaders, as well as by the needs of the community.

Notwithstanding, the focus on reintegration into communities, marriage, families and employment may decrease vulnerability by establishing valuable social ties to institutions and networks – increasing social cohesion in places where societal illnesses such as drug use and HIV may affect social disintegration. Social integration and cohesion can be important in shaping the levels of agency of individuals as well as the structures and institutions in extremely marginalised populations.

The idea that religious institutions can garner support from the state was an important finding. From our discourse analysis and case studies, there are several questions for further research that emerge. Should the state pass some responsibility for the reduction of drug use and HIV infection to religious organisations, considering their possible use of ideological indoctrination? Can institutions, such as FBOs and DRC run by evangelical religious leaders, reduce the vulnerabilities stigma associate with HIV and AIDS if there is greater state and public health collaboration? In part, the state has been efficient at 'delegating' responsibility to civil society in providing such services, even incentivising the growth of civil society networks. When not shaped by the public commitment and control that state affiliation tends to promote, as shown in the case studies, religious moralist and dogmatic discourses and practices may increase the vulnerability of drug users by disregarding human rights, increasing stigmatisation, inhibiting condom use, etc. Analysing the local impacts of a global phenomenon provides a window into the complexities in the responses of civil society and the state to drug use and HIV, especially in countries where the intervention of the state may be limited by economic scarcity and sociocultural marginalisation.

Acknowledgements

This article is based on data collected from the research study titled "Religious Responses to HIV/AIDS in Brazil", a project sponsored by the Eugene Kennedy Shiver US National Institute of Child Health and Human Development (grant number R01 HD050118-05; principal investigator, Richard G. Parker). This national study is being conducted in four sites, at the following institutions and by their respective coordinators: Rio de Janeiro (Associação Brasileira Interdisciplinar de AIDS/ABIA – Veriano Terto Jr.); São Paulo (Universidade de São Paulo/USP – Vera Paiva); Porto Alegre (Universidade Federal do Rio Grande do Sul/ UFRGS – Fernando Seffner); and Recife (Universidade Federal de Pernambuco/UFPE – Luís Felipe Rios). Additional information about the project can be obtained via email from religiao@abiaids.org.br or at http://www.abiaids.org.br, the Associação Brasileira Interdiciplinar de AIDS (ABIA) website.

Jonathan Garcia was supported by F31 HD055153-02 from the Eugene Kennedy Shiver US National Institute of Child Health and Human Development and by T32MH020031 from the National Institute of Mental Health. The content is solely the responsibility of the authors and does not necessarily represent the official views of the NICHD, NIMH or the NIH. Support from the scientists at the Center for Interdisciplinary Research on AIDS at Yale University and the Center for Gender, Sexuality and Health was very valuable in revisions.

Notes

1. In Brazil, there has been a growth of evangelical religions (from 9% in 1991 to 15% in 2000) and a diminishing number of Catholics (from 83% in 1991 to 73% in 2000), according to census data (IBGE 2000). These groups include historical protestant churches, such as Baptists, Presbyterians and Lutherans. Pentecostal groups include groups such as the Assembly of God, the Quadrangular Church, the Universal Church of the Kingdom of God and numerous churches and missions with unique names and followings.
2. The study was approved by the Columbia University Institutional Review Board (IRB), the Committee of Research Ethics of the State University of Rio de Janeiro (CEP/UERJ), as well as by the Brazilian National Research Ethics Commission (CONEP).

References

Adogame, A., 2007. HIV/AIDS support and African Pentecostalism. *Journal of Health Psychology*, 12 (3), 475–484.

Ayres, J.R., 1996. *HIV/AIDS, DST e Abuso de Drogas entre Adolescentes: Vulnerabilidade Avaliação de Ações Preventivas* [HIV/AIDS, STDs and drug abuse in adolescents: vulnerability evaluation and preventive action]. São Paulo: Casa de Edição.

Ayres, J., França Júnior, I., Calazans, G.J., and Saletti Filho, H.C., 2003. O conceito de vulnerabilidade e as práticas de saúde: novas perspectivas e desafios [The vulnerability concept and the practices of health: new perspectives and challenges]. *In*: D. Czeresnia and C.M. Freitas, eds. *Promoção da saúde: conceitos, reflexões, tendências* [Health promotion: concepts, reflections, and tendencies]. Rio de Janeiro: FIOCRUZ, 117–139.

Ayres, J.R.C.M., Paiva, V., França Jr., I., Gravato, N., Lacerda, R., Della Negra, M., Marques, H.H.S., Galano, E., Lecussan, P., and Segurado, A.A.C., 2006. Vulnerability, human rights, and comprehensive care needs of Young people living with HIV/AIDS. *American Journal of Public Health*, 96 (6), 1001–1006.

Azevedo, R.C.S., Botega, N.J., and Guimarães, L.A.M., 2007. Crack users, sexual behavior and HIV infection. *Revista Brasileira de Psiquiatria*, 29 (1), 26–30.

Bastos, F.I., 2009. *Taxas de Infecção de HIV e sífilis e inventário do conhecimento, atitudes e práticas de riscos relacionados às infecções sexualmente transmissíveis entre usuários de drogas em 10 municípios brasileiros* [Rate of infection of HIV and syphilis and inventory of knowledge, attitudes and practices of risk related to sexually transmitted infections in drug users in 10 Brazilian Municipalities]. Technical Report. Brasília: Department of STDs/ AIDS and Viral Hepititis.

Bourdieu, P., 1979. Symbolic power. *Critique of Anthropology*, 4, 77–85.

Brazilian Ministry of Health, 2008. *Epidemiological Bulletin*, V(1) [online]. Available from: http://www.aids.gov.br/data/documents/storedDocuments/%7BB8EF5DAF-23AE-4891-AD36-1903553A3174%7D/%7B31A56BC6-307D-4C88-922D-6F52338D0BF4%7D/Boletim2008_vers%E3o1_6.pdf [Accessed 18 October 2009].

Burdick, J., 1993. *Looking for God in Brazil*. Berkeley and Los Angeles: University of California Press.

Cano, I., 1999. *Letalidade da Ação Policial no Rio de Janeiro: A Atuação da Justiça Militar* [Lethality and police action in Rio de Janeiro: the actions of the military police]. Rio de Janeiro: ISER.

Chesnut, R.A., 1997. *Born again in Brazil: the Pentecostal boom and the pathogens of poverty*. Piscataway, NJ: Rutgers University Press.

Chesnut, R.A., 2003. *Competitive spirits: Latin America's new religious economy.* Oxford: Oxford University Press.

CIDE (Centro de Informações e Dados de Rio de Janeiro), 2005. *Baixada Fluminense em dados* [Baixada Fluminense in data] [online]. Available from: http://www.cide.rj.gov.br/secao.php?secao=4.1 [Accessed 12 October 2008].

Delor, F. and Huber, M., 2000. Revisiting the concept of 'vulnerability'. *Social Science and Medicine,* 50, 1557–1570.

Deng, R., Li, J., Sringernyuang, L., and Zhang, K., 2007. Drug abuse, HIV/AIDS and stigmatisation in a Dai community in Yunnan, China. *Social Science and Medicine,* 64 (8), 1560–1571.

Eriksson, E.L., Lindmark, G., Axemo, P., Haddad, B., and Ahlberg, B.M., 2010. Ambivalence, silence and gender differences in church leaders' HIV-prevention messages to young people in KwaZulu-Natal, South Africa. *Culture Health and Sexuality,* 12 (1), 103–114.

Garcia, J., Muñoz-Laboy, M., de Almeida, V., and Parker, R., 2009. Local impacts of religious discourses on rights to express same-sex sexual desires in peri-urban Rio de Janeiro. *Sexuality Research and Social Policy,* 6 (3), 44–60.

Garcia, M.L.T. and Siqueira, M.M., 2005. Specialized institutions in drug dependence in the state of Espírito Santo. *Jornal Brasileiro de Psiquiatria,* 54 (3), 192–196.

Glaser, B.G. and Strauss, A., 1967. *Discovery of grounded theory: strategies for qualitative research.* Chicago: Aldine.

Hansen, H., 2004. Faith-based treatment for addiction in Puerto Rico. *JAMA,* 291 (23), 2882.

Human Rights Watch, 2009. *Lethal force: police violence and public security in Rio de Janeiro and São Paulo* [online]. Available from: http://www.hrw.org/sites/default/files/reports/brazil1209webwcover.pdf [Accessed 7 February 2011].

Hunt, S., 2000. Winning ways': globalisation and the impact of the health and wealth gospel. *Journal of Contemporary Religion,* 15 (3), 331–347.

IBGE (Instituto Brasileira de Geografia Estatística), 2000. *Censo 2000* [Census 2000] [online]. Available from: http://www.ibge.gov.br/ [Accessed 4 May 2009].

Isham, J., Kelly, K., and Ramaswamy, S., eds., 2002. *Social capital and economic development: well-being in developing countries.* Northampton, MA: Edward Elgar Publishing.

Kawachi, I. and Berkman, L., 2000. *Social epidemiology.* New York: Oxford University Press.

Mann, J. and Tarantola, D., 1996. *AIDS in the world II.* New York: Oxford University Press.

Martins, S., 2004. Vítimas de violência policial se unem contra impunidade [Victims of police violence unite against impunity]. *Jornal Irohin,* 10 [online]. Available from: http://www.irohin.org.br/imp/n10/01a.htm [Accessed 12 December 2008].

Nadanvosky, P., Celeste, R.K., Wilson, M., and Daly, M., 2009. Homicide and impunity: an ecological analysis at state level in Brazil. *Revista de Saúde Pública,* 43 (5), 733–742.

Paim, J.S. and Filho, N.A., 1988. Saúde coletiva: Uma 'nova saúde pública' ou campo aberto a novos paradigmas? [Collective health: a new public health or field for open paradigms?]. *Revista de Saúde Pública,* 32 (4), 299–316.

Pechansky, F., Woody, G., Inciardi, J., Surratt, H., Kessler, F., Von Diemen, L., and Bumaguin, D., 2006. HIV seroprevalence among drug users: an analysis of selected variables based on 10 years of data collection in Porto Alegre, Brazil. *Drug and Alcohol Dependence,* 82, S109–S113.

Sanchez, Z.V.D.M. and Nappo, S.A., 2008. Religious treatments for drug addiction: an exploratory study in Brazil. *Social Science and Medicine,* 67, 638–646.

Smith, D.J., 2004. Youth, sin and sex in Nigeria: Christianity and HIV/AIDS-related beliefs and behaviour among rural-urban migrants. *Culture, Health and Sexuality,* 6 (5), 425–437.

Soares, L.E., 1996. *Violência e política no Rio de Janeiro* [Violence and politics in Rio de Janeiro]. Rio de Janeiro: Relume-Dumará.

Szwarcwald, C.L., Bastos, F.I., Barcellos, C., de Fátima Pina, M., and Pires Esteves, M.A., 2000. Health conditions and residential concentration of poverty: a study in Rio de Janeiro, Brazil. *Journal of Epidemiology and Community Health,* 54, 530–536.

Todd, C.S., Nassiramenesh, B., Stanekzai, M.R., and Kamarulzaman, A., 2007. Emerging HIV epidemics in Muslim countries: assessment of different cultural responses to harm reduction and implications for HIV control. *Current HIV/AIDS Reports,* 4 (4), 151–157.

Blood, sweat and semen: The economy of *axé* and the response of Afro-Brazilian religions to HIV and AIDS in Recife

Luis Felipe Rios[a], Cinthia Oliveira[a], Jonathan Garcia[b], Miguel Muñoz-Laboy[c], Laura Murray[c] and Richard Parker[c,d]

[a]Laboratory for the Study of Human Sexuality, Universidade Federal de Pernambuco, Recife, Brazil; [b]Center for Interdisciplinary Research on AIDS, Yale School of Public Health, Yale University, New Haven, CT, USA; [c]Department of Sociomedical Sciences, Columbia University, New York, NY, USA; [d]ABIA, Rio de Janeiro, Brazil

This article provides an ethnographic analysis of Afro-Brazilian religious responses to the HIV epidemic in Recife. Drawing on participant observation and in-depth interviews conducted with Afro-Brazilian religious leaders and public health officials, it highlights the importance of the *axé* – a mystical energy manipulated in religious rituals that is symbolically associated with blood, sweat and semen. In an analysis of the relationship formed between the state AIDS programme and Afro-Brazilian religious centres, we conclude that the recognition of native categories and their meanings is one of the key elements to a fruitful dialogue between public health programmes and religious leaders that in the case studied, resulted in the re-signification of cultural practices to prevent HIV. Although the Afro-Brazilian religious leaders interviewed tended to be more open about sexuality and condom promotion, stigma towards people living with HIV (PLHIV) was still present within the religious temples, yet appeared to be more centred upon the perception of HIV as negatively affecting followers' *axé* than judgement related to how one may have contracted the virus. We discuss the tensions between taking a more liberal and open stance on prevention, while also fostering attitudes that may stigmatise PLHIV, and make suggestions for improving the current Afro-Brazilian response to the epidemic.

Introduction

Brazil is especially well known for the effectiveness of its response to HIV and AIDS. Its National AIDS Programme is widely recognised as one of the leading AIDS prevention and control programmes in the world (Berkman *et al.* 2005, Okie 2006), and the interaction between civil society and the Brazilian government has been identified as a key element in building the Brazilian response to the epidemic as a model for other developing countries (Berkman *et al.* 2005). From the very beginning of the epidemic, religious leaders and institutions from diverse denominations have been central to the Brazilian response to the AIDS epidemic (Galvão 1997). However, to date, there has been little recognition of the fact that organised religion, religious beliefs and religious institutions and organisations have played a key role in shaping the country's response.

In order to respond to this gap, an extensive, comparative multi-site ethnographic study was conducted between 2005 and 2010 in Rio de Janeiro, São Paulo (both in the south-east of Brazil), Porto Alegre (in the south) and Recife (in the north-east). The overall study was designed to document the ways in which the Roman Catholic Church, Evangelical Protestant and Afro-Brazilian religious traditions have contributed to the broader social response to HIV and AIDS in Brazil. This paper analyses the engagement of Afro-Brazilian religions in responding to the HIV epidemic in Recife. We focus on the specific cultural symbols and practices that affected the vulnerability of religious followers to HIV transmission and HIV related stigma. Our discussion is organised in four parts. First, we expound on the notion of *axé* (a mystical energy manipulated in religious rituals that is symbolically associated with blood, sweat and semen), focusing on its interactions with corporeal phenomenon and providing the necessary background on Afro-Brazilian religions to understand how the *terreiros*, or places of worship, became involved in the Brazilian response to HIV and AIDS. After providing this contextual background, we analyse the narratives of Afro-Brazilian religious priests and public health officials to understand the reasons why they became involved in HIV prevention and have an apparently more open approach to prevention discourses than other religious leaders interviewed in the larger study, yet also appear to hold stigmatising beliefs towards people living with HIV (PLHIV). We end considering possible paths to improve the quality of the current Afro-Brazilian response to the epidemic.

Afro-Brazilian religions in Brazil

The history of Afro-Brazilian religions in Brazil, similar to many religions in countries of the African Diaspora, can be traced back to communal resistance against the violent conditions of slavery. In contrast to the *quilombos*, independent settlements of runaway slaves, Afro-Brazilian religions provided a platform for organised resistance (Vogel *et al.* 1993). Even though they were strongly contested, the religious ideology was very successful, and today a variety of beliefs that originated from Afro-Brazilian religions are offered as spiritual paths not only for Blacks, but also for men and women from a variety of sociocultural, racial and ethnic groups (Prandi 1991).

In the 2000 Brazilian census, only 0.34% of the population declared themselves to be practitioners of Afro-Brazilian religions, yet it is difficult to estimate the exact number of followers for several reasons. First, there is a strong history of persecution of followers, which has led to reluctance to self-identify with the religion as one's primary religious affiliation. In recent years, Afro-Brazilian religious deities have been demonised by the neo-Pentecostals (a rapidly growing population in Brazil). In the face of widespread stigmatisation, many followers prefer to say they are Catholic (73.8% of respondents on the 2000 census) or Kardecist Spiritualism (1.3% on the 2000 census) – both religious denominations that are perceived as being more respected (Instituto Brasileira de Geografia Estatística [IBGE] 2000, Prandi 2004). A second, and related reason is that the strong tradition of religious syncretism in Brazil has made it possible for people to identify with more than one religion. Thus, replying that one is Catholic in the census does not conflict with practicing aspects of Afro-Brazilian religions as well. The pervasiveness of Afro-Brazilian religious traditions in Brazil can be most visibly seen in the ubiquitous presence of Afro-Brazilian religious deities in popular culture and many of Brazil's festivals (Pierruci and Prandi 2000). Thus, while the actual percentage of people identifying exclusively with the Afro-Brazilian religious traditions is low, the influence of the religions on Brazilian life is generally considered to be quite high.

There are diverse denominations within the Afro-Brazilian religious traditions that are historically each tied to distinct regions of the country. Academic literature links *Candomblé* to Bahia and Rio de Janeiro, *Xangô* and *Jurema* to Recife, *Batuque* to Porto Alegre, and *Umbanda* to Rio de Janeiro and São Paulo. The specific social and cultural processes through which the denominations have evolved over time are complex, and for the purposes of this study, we categorised the various denominations in the four cities studied into two large matrices: (1) Africanist religions that aim for a greater proximity with African cultures – *Xangô, Candomblé* and *Batuque* and (2) religions that mix elements of Catholicism with indigenous and African religions – *Umbanda* and *Jurema* (Silva 1994, Rios 2000, Bastide 2001, Prandi 2001a, Brandão and Rios 2002).[1]

In this article, we focus our analysis on the Africanist religions *Candomblé* and *Xangô*, since they were the first ones the government HIV and AIDS programmes approached to be involved in prevention activities in Brazil. As will be described in detail below, the government first approached religious leaders due to the techniques of bodily scarification used during initiation rituals that involved the sharing of non-sterilised cutting instruments, and the strong presence of people with homosexual practices, who are one of the population groups in Brazil most vulnerable to HIV infection.

Research setting and methodology

The field research was conducted between 2005 and 2007 in the metropolitan region of Recife, Brazil. Recife is the capital of Pernambuco State, the fastest-growing urban area in north-eastern Brazil, with a population of roughly 3,750,000. Metropolitan Recife is considered the origin of *Xangô* and *Jurema*, however after the 1960s, the appearance of *Candomblé* and *Umbanda* diversified the religious landscape (Rios 2000). The exact number of *terreiros* is unknown, but the strong presence of these religions is obvious nonetheless, especially in the urban periphery.

The research involved participant observation in places of worship for the different traditions, as well as AIDS related activities sponsored by the National Network of Afro-Brazilian Religions and Health[2] (Garcia and Parker 2011) and the Pernambuco State and City of Recife Departments of Health. Field notes were written daily, providing a 'thick description' (Geertz 1973) of the events observed. In addition, we conducted a total of 28 interviews with 19 people, including nine with Afro-Brazilian religious priests – three from *Umbanda*, two from *Candomblé* (*Keto* and *Angola* nations), three from *Xangô* (*Xambá* and *Nagô* nations) and one from *Jurema* – as well as 10 representatives of governmental and nongovernmental organisations involved in religious mobilisation against AIDS. The priests all participated in both a life history and oral history interview, and the representatives from governmental and nongovernmental organisations all participated in an in-depth interview. Numerous informal conversations with religious individuals and several professionals who worked together with the *terreiros* in response to the HIV epidemic were also considered a resource for data collection. The study was approved by the Brazilian Research Ethics Commission (CONEP) and the Institutional Review Board of Columbia University Medical Center.

We took an inductive approach to the analysis of interview transcripts and fieldnotes to allow for the emergence of 'emic' categories and an exploration of culture in practice (Sahlins 2000). While the analytical categories were grounded in the terminology used by the participants, theoretical frameworks that emphasise the sociocultural construction of corporal events (Foucault 1976, 2008, Le Breton 2006) guided our analysis.

Afro-Brazilian religious practices and HIV

Candomblé and Xangô are considered polytheistic religions because they have multiple deities, called *orixás*. The high point of the religious ceremonies is when the *orixás* become present through possession, often receiving sacrificial animals that are prepared in accordance with sacred recipes and then shared among the community. The ceremonies occur in *terreiros*, or temples, that exist to enable favourable contact between *aiê* (the world, inhabited by humans) and *orun* (the other world, inhabited by divine beings) and are organised around a hierarchical structure that mimics a familial context. Each *terreiro* has a *pai* or *mãe de santo* (literally the father or mother of the saint), who takes on the role of the supreme priest and is assisted by other priests called the *filhos de santo* (children of the saint). In order to have access to the most sacred of the religious knowledge, and be a medium for the *orixás*, the children of the saint must be ordained through initiation rituals that in very general terms involves the passing of *axé,* loosely translated to mean the energy that is the source of life. According to native beliefs, *axé* has many qualities that are closely related to natural elements and phenomena (water, fire, storms, rocks, etc.) and can be accumulated, transmitted and lost. Wherever it moves, or flows, it transmits traces of where it was previously. In this way, if *axé* is first considered to be an undifferentiated energy that gives life to the world, when it is manipulated and passed on through ceremonies in the *terreiros*, it is modified and imprinted with traces of the *terreiros* in the process. It is through this process – the transfer and modification of *axé* – that its meaning and importance in the Afro-Brazilian religious tradition emerges.

On the individual level, each person receives a specific amount and type of *axé* to secure their existence in the world. But, throughout one's life, the quantity and kind of *axé* they have is understood to vary and be influenced by specific bodily and social practices. For example, disease, suffering and fatigue occur when *axé* diminishes, and when the *axé* is plentiful, it can increase prosperity in all areas of one's life. Religious practices seek to intervene and redirect the flow and accumulation of positive *axé* through rituals that connect this world with the other world by tapping into ethereal resources (Barros and Teixeira 1989, Rios 2004).

In the initiation rituals, small cuts are made in specific parts of the initiate's body (on top of one's head and shoulders) to permit the entrance of substances prepared in accordance with the precepts of *terreiro* to pass on the sacred energy. The parts of the body with cuts are then sprinkled with the blood of the sacrificial animals. The animal blood is considered to be a vehicle for *axé*, and it is through the ritual that the *axé* of the *terreiro's* religious tradition is considered to enter into the initiate.

In Afro-Brazilian religious beliefs, the *axé* takes on a tangible nature, such as the substances used on the ritual cuts and bodily fluids. It is through contact with these tangible substances that the energy passes from one being to another. Therefore, in addition to the blood of the sacrificial animals, the sweat for example that drops from the priest's face onto the heads of the *orixá*'s dearest acolytes while he is in a trance for an *orixá* is understood to bring those who receive it several gains. *Axé* can also be transferred in settings outside of the *terreiro*, and followers believe that semen can transfers *axé* from person to person during sexual intercourse.

The process of passing *axé* is of particular interest to this research and public health officials due to the specific beliefs surrounding the passing of *axé* during sex and the tools often used in the initiation rituals, such as the razors. In *Candomblé* and *Xangô*, when granted permission from the *orixás* to initiate new sons or daughters, the priest receives a razor (among other objects) as a signal that she/he is authorised to be a *pai* or *mãe de santo*. The razor is used to open ritual cuts through which the *axé* of the *terreiro* can enter into bodies of the followers. Prior to the arrival of public health officials in the *terreiros*, religious precepts stipulated that the *pai* or *mãe de santo* use the same razor to scar all of their children. Many people often participated in scarification rituals together, and were all cut by the same razor which was never properly sterilised (i.e., in accordance with public health guidelines) between cuts. Razors were seen as being imbued with *axé* throughout the religious rituals that occurred in the *terreiro* over time, and the collective use of the same razor blade during initiation rituals was understood to be a way to pass on the *axés* of the religious community to the initiates.

The sharing of the razors is what first brought the Pernambuco AIDS Programme to the *terreiros* in Recife. Rather than altering the initiation rituals, the AIDS programme sought to encourage the use of disposable razors. At first, it was difficult for the priests to consider changing their practices, as the nature of repeated use of the razors was precisely what gave them value for the initiation rituals. *Pai* João[3] detailed the difficulties he first faced when the state AIDS programme approached him:

> 'So we [priests] realised that the razor could be a tool that would lead and/or contribute to increasing AIDS in the communities. It was not easy for us to alter our practices... [people said] "This razor is the razor that came from my grandfather, then everyone has to go through it!" It was a matter of tradition'. (*Pai* João, 68 years, *Xangô*)

It is important to emphasise that it is not because of 'religious ignorance' that the priest would affirm, 'I will not switch [razors], no!'. It is due to the power that the priest attributed to the razor as a conductor of *axé*. The cuts made in the scarification rituals form an essential element in the sociocultural reproduction in *Xangô* and *Candomblé*, and the biomedical discourse of the AIDS programme calling for the use of disposable razors was initially seen as threatening the *terreiro* tradition.

The Secretary of Health formed a working group with religious leaders as a way to reflect on the health implications of reusing the ritual razors. Concerned about the consequences of switching razors, the leaders decided to search for more information about the initiation ritual and conducted their own historical research regarding the cutting instruments used for scarification. As *Pai* João explains:

> 'Because, after thorough research, we did not find any book or African history, saying that the German razor was the only instrument that could be used. At that time, the first razors were German. (...) The razor appeared solely as an instrument that was good for cutting. The barber shaved his beard, and this led the *pai* of the *terreiro* to understand that it was good to shave the beard and the head and make the cuts. Today we work with a disposable razor; it is not possible to do otherwise'. (*Pai* João)

When they discovered that over time the instruments used for scarification had changed, the religious leaders were able to shift the meaning of the razor. They reduced the importance of the razor as a conductor of *axé*, and instead agreed that its most important function was its ability to cut. This brought about an important change: the individualisation of the razor used in initiation rituals and/or its sterilisation in accordance with medical guidelines.

Sex and the terreiros

When comparing Afro-Brazilian religions to other religions in Brazilian society, academic studies tend to present them as more permissive when it comes to sexual morality – in particular, in their openness to homosexualities.[4] Still, studies suggest that even though the sex-gender system of the *terreiros* does not emphasise regulation of followers' sex lives in accordance with heteronormative values, rules and regulations situated within the very logic of the *axé* still exist (Barros and Teixeira 1989, Segato 1995, Rios 2004).

For example, participation in some religious services is dependent on following a series of sexual restrictions. Research participants recognised the repressive nature of some of these restrictions:

> '... the Orixá forbids you to do certain things. Among those things are to go to the [prostitution] zone, for example. (...) To hit on a lady [prostitute], because he knows that the woman takes over his body ... and he is a bit startled with that and he fears that the deity will punish him too. Because he went to such an environment ... with drinks ... menstruating women, sick women (...) an environment where, for us, there is negative energy. So there are many people who will not go, they are afraid they'll get negative energy. *Candomblé* contributes precisely with this repression. Let's say, it's ... prevention, not repression, but prevention: 'You will not go because you can get sick'-that is to prevent!' (*Pai* João)

Several of our interviewees identified the sexual norms of the *terreiros* as affecting their prevention activities. *Pai* João, in the quote above, centred his rationale for avoiding prostitution zones on the notion of a dirty body and a clean body (Barros and Teixeira 1989, Rios 2004). A clean body is associated with positive energy, a requirement to participate in the rituals. Having a dirty body in a ritual is considered by our interviewees as a form of serious misconduct, as stated by *Pai* João:

> 'It is about sin. When it is about sin, it upsets God. You only sin when you act against the divine, when you act against the orixá, isn't it so? In our religion, if you have sex,

you cannot participate in the ritual (...) the person has a dirty body! A dirty soul'. (*Pai* João)

Thus, according to the discourse of *Pai* João, the dangers of 'energy contamination' from prostitutes leads some men to avoid areas of prostitution and is also seen as contributing to the prevention of HIV by avoiding what they perceive to be risky sexual encounters.

Although the priests discuss rules regulating sexuality, they also recognise the existence of 'free will'. In their narratives, the concept of the 'flesh' appears in relation to the concept of 'choice' and is synonymous with sexual desire and provocative behaviour. Such behaviours are referred to as going against the prescribed sexual mores of the *terreiros* and of the broader society and often contributing to unplanned pregnancy and the spread of HIV. When asked about the capacity of individuals to follow religious precepts on sexuality, *Pai* João explained why there is a disconnect between the religious ideal and what actually happens (i.e., pollution of the body):

'Because the flesh does not know obedience! The flesh does not respect anything or anyone! If the flesh rules, it happens at any time, at any place and at any age!' (*Pai* João)

Although dangerous (because it can lead the individual to make mistakes), the flesh in the context of Afro-Brazilian religions is also spoken about positively in relation to pleasure. Religious mythologies present it as a natural part of the fecundity and fertility of individuals and as being positively associated with bodily pleasure (Prandi 2001b). In their narratives, interviewees recognised the power of the flesh, yet also emphasised the importance of managing sexual desire responsibly:

[In response to a question about the ideal time to start one's sexual life] 'From the time he starts to take responsibility for things. (...) I believe that 40% of 18 year old youngsters, in that range, have responsibility. Responsibility to their family. "Well, my father said so, so I will obey". Others have responsibility to their girlfriends, to the family of the girlfriend, and others have a responsibility to themselves: "I cannot do it because I cannot assume a child"; "I do not want to spoil my studies"; "I do not want to do this, I do not want to do that ..." It's called responsibility!' (*Pai* João)

Thus, summarising the interviews with *Pai* João and our other Afro-Brazilian religious interviewees, responsibility is an achievement in personal development, an internalisation of social knowledge and norms. Problems and possible contamination are seen as being associated with irresponsibly following one's will. Being responsible and knowledgeable about the consequences of sexual actions are perceived as protecting and keeping oneself safe. Another *Pai de santo* describes it as follows:

[From your point of view, or even in the religion, when and under what circumstances should the youngsters start their sexual life?] 'I think it's from the time he is secure. He is secure, he is aware, he has guidance. I think sex is not a bad thing, right? I think it is even good! But I think for that to happen, one must know what they want with a partner and really see what he/she is doing, right? Orientation, seeking always to talk with their parents, who are the friendliest persons who can guide them ... Being safe, really, and seeing what is good for him/her. And if she knows that, she will prevent AIDS, know how to wear a condom, if she does not want to use, she asks her partner to use, to prevent a pregnancy and a disease, right? And an unwanted pregnancy, to prevent future suffering...' (*Pai* Claudio)

Pai João and *Pai* Claudio tell us about the need to be responsible and secure as a way to prevent adverse consequences associated with the pleasures of the flesh. The concept of 'security' is closely related to an idea of being safe from unwanted pregnancy, HIV and suffering. In research conducted as part of the larger research project with Catholics and evangelical Protestants, 'responsibility' and 'security' also emerged as protective devices (Rios *et al.* 2008). For Afro-Brazilians, responsibility is understood as a way to discipline the flesh. In the context of HIV prevention and treatment programmes within which this research was conducted, the priests' discourses surrounding responsibility and security as key components to upholding social norms and maintaining health overlap with contemporary biomedical discourses of risk (Caliman 2006, Foucault 2008). Responsibility and safety thus emerge as categories where religious and public health beliefs coincide and open up space for collaboration.

Pai Claudio's speech eloquently defines what might be considered similar to the security mechanisms described by Foucault (2008) that operate in conjunction with technologies of biopower to organise one's future material and spiritual possibilities in a way that ultimately upholds larger systems of power. Religious followers' decisions to avoid sex or the prostitution zone are examples of security mechanisms that reinforce and reproduce religious and biomedical discourses and are employed in hopes that they will result in good health and please the *orixás*.

In our research, Catholic, Evangelical and Afro-Brazilian religious leaders discussed responsibility and security not only in the context of contemporary biomedical discourses surrounding 'risk', but also in relation to the social and cultural context within which their followers live. In interviews, they frequently referred to the way in which sexuality permeates non-religious institutions and ideologies. In particular, they referred to images and sexual ideas in the media:

'I am against the TV show *Malhação*,[5] and I'll explain why. In *Malhação*, you see girls starting their sexual life with their boyfriends. I am partly in favour and partly against this [the programme]. Because it is a consumer product that goes into one's house ... and enters the home of some girl, who lives in a poor place, in a slum. And when the same girl is with her sweetheart, we cannot judge, but her thinking is guided more below the belt, so to say, and ends up having sex with him. After she has sex with him, he also has no maturity...' (*Pai* Fernando)

Pai Fernando's narrative highlights the changing social environment within which individuals are perceived to negotiate both modern secular and religious ideals (Berger and Luckman 1966). Youth, for example, are perceived to receive messages from the media, their families and religions and then negotiate their boundaries and 'risks' individually. 'Responsible' youth are those who weigh their risks and make the 'safest' decisions that will protect them from threats like unwanted pregnancy and HIV. Religious youth must also consider the spiritual consequences to their actions, and are expected to make responsible decisions that will lead to their sexual *and* spiritual health.

Public health response to AIDS in Recife

Brazil's solidarity and citizenship approach to HIV prevention, with a focus on promoting condoms and working in partnership with civil society (Governo do Brasil n/d, Parker 2003), facilitated the development of positive relationships with religious leaders. In Pernambuco, the relationship began when the state STD/AIDS Programme sought out the *terreiros* due to concerns with razor blade use in the initiation rituals. In acknowledging both the limits of religious discipline in 'protecting' followers from AIDS and the dangers, and pleasures, of sex, all the Afro-Brazilian priests and priestesses interviewed recognised the importance of collaborating with public HIV prevention programmes. In interviews, priests and priestesses mentioned having come in contact with PLHIV in their *terreiros* prior to implementing interventions; yet the partnership with the state HIV programme marked the first time that Afro-Brazilian religious leaders formally committed to systematically working on HIV and AIDS.

In 2000, a taskforce was formed involving *pais* and *mães de santo*, anthropologists, and State Health Secretariat specialists to think about actions to combat the epidemic in the *terreiros*. In the beginning, the task force primarily focused on preventing HIV transmission through sharp instruments, distributing an educational booklet (Revista Atotô 2001) and touring several *terreiros* to give lectures. Although the edition of the booklet is no longer in print, several interviewees cited that the workshops organised by the state health secretariat and the municipal STD/AIDS coordination in Recife for religious leaders are still occurring.

As *Pai* Claudio recounts below, priests recognised the difficulties they faced when they first started addressing the issue:

> [Do you remember what the first meeting was like?] 'The first one was not very good, right? The first one was not very good ... I had little knowledge and I conveyed very little to them, right? I invited many who did not come. [Many said] "Ah! I do not want to know, pai, about these things! I do not have AIDS, nothing is wrong with me". And I'd say, "that's what I'm telling you, thank God you don't have anything. But you have to learn now, in order not to get it". Yeah, you know, there was little knowledge, and then it got better. And nowadays it's much better. They [followers] talk about it [AIDS] nowadays ... sometimes, they come talk to me'. (*Pai* Claudio)

Pai Claudio's narrative points both to the ways in which his knowledge and understanding of AIDS evolved, and how this affected his relationship with members of the *terreiro*. Over time, he came to be seen as a resource for information and support about HIV, in addition to distributing prevention supplies such as condoms. Distributing condoms, especially to young people, was often mentioned in interviews as part of supporting youth's sense of responsibility and safety.

In interviews, priests and public health officials esteemed their relationship as fruitful because of their success in making it possible for *terreiros* to engage in prevention. Razor use and sexuality were mentioned as being openly discussed and informative materials were distributed within the *terreiros* themselves – something less common in some Catholic or Evangelical churches in Recife, where abstinence for single people and fidelity for married people were the primary forms of prevention openly supported by the religious leaders (Rios *et al.* 2008).

Although Brazil's constitution guarantees universal access to health care, including prevention and free treatment, and the Ministry of Health emphasises the right of PLHIV to live in a community free of prejudice and discrimination, PLHIV often face stigma due to their HIV status, that can be even more pronounced in some religious settings. In observing the different initiatives of the *terreiros*, we did not see or hear anything specific related to the stigmatisation of PLHIV. However, as we explore further below, beliefs surfaced in interviews surrounding HIV that were consistent with Afro-Brazilian viewpoints towards the negative aspects of sickness.

Axé, HIV and stigma

Discourses referring to being able to cure AIDS were absent from the priest and priestesses' narratives, yet they did emphasise the role of religion in offering spiritual comfort to those living with HIV. However, only one of those interviewed mentioned having HIV-positive *filhos de santo* in their *terreiros*. More common were remarks about their presence in other *terreiros* and the potential negative impact of having PLHIV in the *terreiro*. The virtual invisibility of PLHIV in the Afro-Brazilian *terreiros* may be related to stigma. As *Pai* Joao states:

> 'Yes, there is discrimination, indeed! Absolutely. The terreiros... I believe that if you have a pai de santo with AIDS, there are few people who would attend his house, client or filho de santo, for sure. They go away, for sure'. (Pai Joao)

The invisibility of PLHIV may then be related to discrimination, which discourages those living with HIV to disclose their status. Another possibility is that the priests, conscious of the stigma towards HIV, avoid sharing any knowledge of HIV positive followers in their *terreiros*.

The discrimination mentioned towards PLHIV is closely related to the Afro-Brazilian religious tradition's beliefs that disease signals the decline of *axé*. Although the way in which sickness is treated differs slightly in the distinct matrices of the religious traditions, for the Africanists in which this research is focused, the main purpose of the *terreiro* is to have a space to cultivate a relationship with the deities. Sicknesses treated within the *terreiro* are primarily those that are perceived as being in some way a punishment from the deities. Since *axé* in the Africanist belief system relies on a conductor to pass it from one to another, it is possible that the discrimination referred to in our interviews is connected to a belief that if a *pai* or *mãe de santo* was HIV positive, they would not be able to pass *axé* (representing life) onto another person because they would be understood to be contaminated with HIV (representative of death). Another concern is that in the rituals, if it were understood that the presence of PLHIV could influence the passage of *axé*, this could also contribute towards the stigma and discrimination of PLHIV.

More research is needed to explore the connections between beliefs surrounding *axé*, HIV and stigma in the Afro-Brazilian religions, yet some ethnographic studies have found that *terreiros* lose their *filhos de santo* when the leader becomes ill (Brandão 1990, Carvalho 2000). For example, in his book on HIV-positive religious figures and the impact of HIV on their religious trajectories, Carvalho (2000) discusses how the Afro-Brazilian priest they interviewed lost his religious community when he disclosed his HIV status. In informal conversations that emerged during our fieldwork, there was constant reference to priests who lost their *filhos de santo* when they disclosed their HIV status – or of *filhos de santo* who are pushed into more private rituals and forms of worship when their HIV status reaches the ears of their *pais de santo*.

Final considerations for discussion

Several important points emerge from the empirical data collected in Recife. First, the recognition of 'native' categories and their meanings was one of the key elements to a fruitful dialogue between public health programmes and religious leaders. Second, we found that certain cultural practices and understandings were subject to modification. Although the religious structures generally prescribed how people should behave and think, our observations related to the scarification rituals in particular pointed to various reconfigurations, rearticulations and redescriptions in practice (Sahlins 1985) that often reflected some overlap with public health categories of 'responsibility' and 'security'. Finally, we found that although the Afro-Brazilian religious leaders interviewed tended to be more open about sexuality and condom promotion, stigma towards PLHIV was still present within the *terreiros*, yet appeared to be more centred upon the perception of HIV polluting blood/*axé*, than judgement related to how one may have contracted the virus.

The relationship between the state HIV programme and religious groups had important effects that appeared to impact the health of religious followers in several important ways. On one hand, it facilitated the re-signification of scarification, by de-emphasising the blade as a carrier of *axé*, and positioning it instead as a mere 'surgical' instrument that opened the possibility for *axé* to be transmitted. On the other hand, the conception of bodily fluids (sweat, sperm and saliva) as a vehicle of *axé*, combined with the existent controls on sexuality (i.e., discouraging visits to prostitution zones) were understood as protective strategies against personal HIV 'pollution' and however erroneous, made the incorporation of public health prevention technologies, like condoms, easier.

We found that it was the centrality of blood in the symbolism of *axé* and HIV and AIDS that created conditions that reinforced stigma. As Parker and Aggleton demonstrate (2003), the processes of stigmatisation against PLHIV go beyond interfering in the realm of personal illness, to influencing the efficacy of prevention actions and reinforcing other forms of social inequality. PLHIV were not only perceived as losing energy/power due to being sick (or as sick because they lost *axé*), but also as a person that, because they were understood to have polluted blood/*axé*, is also capable of contaminating the entire community. Contamination was understood to occur directly through bodily fluids or simply by coming in contact with someone thought to have 'polluted' blood. The idea of pollution surfaced both in commentaries with respect to HIV and the justifications given for why *filhos de santo* should avoid prostitution zones.

In this context, 'responsibility' and 'safety' emerged as categories in both public health and religious narratives, indicating the existence of a surreptitious dialogue between religious discourse and discourse of the risk peculiar to contemporary medical science (Foucault 2008). In our interpretation, responsibility and safety as categories for promoting protective behaviour also reflect a recognition on behalf of Afro-Brazilian religious leaders of the social and cultural (and secular) context in which their followers live and the futility of attempting to control sexuality. In the context of contemporary liberal Brazilian society, calling for the construction of individual responsibility, connected to the idea of safety, appears to have been a good strategy, along with the distribution of prevention supplies (like razors and condoms) to guarantee *axé* and health.[6]

While the incorporation of blade asepsis and individual razors in rituals and condom distribution appear to have reached some level of success in terms of HIV prevention, our findings point to the need for more research on the experiences of HIV positive followers and priests in Afro-Brazilian *terreiros*, with a focus on the relationship between blood, *axé* and HIV. This research should be carried out within a theoretical context that permits a critical analysis of the cultural shifts in meanings and significations that constitute religious experiences (Sahlins 1985), and the ways in which they overlap and/or depart from contemporary biomedical discourses surrounding HIV. In our research, we found that religious figures have adapted when confronted by HIV, motivated by the need to preserve and protect life. Further anthropological research could provide a fuller understanding of the social and cultural practices and beliefs surrounding HIV, and be used to develop interventions that enable Afro-Brazilian religious groups to reflect on their practices (including their own forms of oppression) and rediscover their role as fundamentally inclusive religions. We conclude by remembering that the *terreiros* were (and still are, in some sense) at the forefront of the inclusion of 'minorities' (Blacks, women, homosexuals, poor people and a whole range of marginalised individuals) in the high ranks of the priestly hierarchies. Their commitment to inclusion, combined with a historical trajectory of transnational cultural transfigurations, has created an openness and flexibility that could also encourage a more inclusive approach to those living with HIV.

Acknowledgements

This article is based on data collected from the study Religious Responses to HIV/AIDS in Brazil, a project sponsored by the US Eunice Kennedy Shriver National Institute of Child Health and Human Development (grant number 1 R01 HD050118; principal investigator, Richard G. Parker). This national study is conducted in four sites, at the following institutions and by their respective coordinators: Rio de Janeiro (Associação Brasileira Interdisciplinar de AIDS/ABIA – Veriano Terto Jr.), São Paulo (Universidade de São Paulo/USP – Vera Paiva), Porto Alegre (Universidade Federal do Rio Grande do Sul/UFRGS – Fernando Seffner) and Recife (Universidade Federal de Pernambuco/ UFPE – Luís Felipe Rios). Additional information about the project can be obtained via e-mail from religiao@abiaids.org.br or at http://www.abiaids.org.br. The content is solely the responsibility of the authors and does not necessarily represent the official views of the Eunice Kennedy Shriver National Institute of Child Health and Human Development or the National Institutes of Health.

Notes

1. One of the major elements of Africanist traditions is the nature of spiritual entities worshiped. While deities and spirits are worshiped in both matrices, in the Africanists matrices, only the deities can incorporate their followers in a trance. In the religions with more Christian influence, the spirits of the dead are understood to be the ones with this power.
2. http://religrafosaude.blogspot.com/
3. To preserve the anonymity of the interviewees we are using fictitious names.

4. Here it is important to remember that male homosexuals were, at the beginning of the epidemic, identified as a risk group and remain one of the populations most vulnerable to HIV. For a review of the debate about homosexuality in the field of Afro-Brazilian studies, see Fry (2010).
5. Soap opera shown in the late afternoon, directed at adolescents and broadcast on one of Brazil's primary television stations.
6. For a more detailed analysis of the relationship between individual risk, security and responsibility in the religious context, see Rios *et al.* (2008).

References

Barros, J. and Teixeira, M.L., 1989. O código do corpo: inscrições do orixás [The code of the body: inscriptions of the *orixás*]. *In*: C. Moura, ed. *Meu sinal está em teu corpo* [My symptom is in your body]. São Paulo: EDICON/EDUSP, 36–42.

Bastide, R., 2001. *O candomblé da Bahia* [The *Candomblé* of Bahia]. São Paulo: Companhia das Letras.

Berger, P. and Luckmann, T., 1966. *The social construction of reality: a treatise in the sociology of knowledge*. Garden City, NY: Anchor Books.

Berkman, A., Garcia, J., Muñoz-Laboy, M., Paiva, V., and Parker, R., 2005. A critical analysis of the Brazilian response to HIV/AIDS: lessons learned for controlling and mitigating the epidemic in developing countries. *American Journal of Public Health*, 95 (7), 1162–1172.

Brandão, M., 1990. O pai e a mãe de santo no sistema de alocação de recursos: agenciamento da chefia religiosa [The father and mother saints in the system of resource distribution: agency of religious leaders]. *Cadernos do mestrado em Antropologia* [Masters theses in Anthropology], 2, 25–36. Recife: Federal University of Pernambuco.

Brandão, M. and Rios, L.F., 2002. El campo religioso afro-recifense contemporâneo: nuevos modelos religiosos y políticas de identidade [The contemporary religious terrain of Afro-Recifenses: new models of religions and political identities]. *In*: J. Monter, ed. *Integración social y cultural* [Cultural and social integration]. Spain: Universidade da Corunã, 53–68.

Caliman, L., 2006. Dominando corpos, conduzindo ações: genealogias do biopoder em Foucault [Dominating bodies, steering actions: geneologies of bio-power in Foucault]. *In*: A.M. Jacó-Vilela, A.C. Cerezzo, and H. Rodrigues, eds. *Clio-Psyché – Subjetividade e História* [Clio-Psyché – Subjectivity and History]. Juiz de Fora: Clio Edições Eletrônicas, 200–211.

Carvalho, C., 2000. *Tessituras de segredos e silêncios: o viver com AIDS* [Sacred and silent structures: living with AIDS]. Masters thesis. Universidade Federal de Pernambuco.

Foucault, M., 1976. *The history of sexuality vol. 1: the will to knowledge*. London: Penguin.

Foucault, M., 2008. *Microfísica do poder* [The microphysics of power]. Rio de Janeiro: Graal.

Fry, P., 2010. Presentation. *Vibrant*, 7 (1), 7–10.

Galvão, J., 1997. As respostas religiosas frente à epidemia de HIV/AIDS no Brasil [Religious responses to the HIV/AIDS epidemic in Brazil]. *In*: R. Parker, ed. *Políticas, instituições e AIDS: enfrentando a epidemia no Brasil* [Politics, institutions and AIDS: confronting the epidemic in Brazil]. Rio de Janeiro: Jorge Zahar/ABIA, 67–108.

Garcia, J. and Parker, R., 2011. Resource mobilization for health advocacy: Afro-Brazilian religious organizations and HIV prevention and control. *Social Science & Medicine*, 72 (12), 1930–1938.

Geertz, C., 1973. *The interpretation of cultures*. New York: Basic Books.

Governo do Brasil, n/d. *Departamento de DST e AIDS* [online]. Available from: http://www.aids.gov.br/main.asp?View={CEBD192A-348E-4E7E-8735-B30000865D1C}&Mode=1 [Accessed 9 January 2009].

Instituto Brasileira de Geografia Estatística, 2000. *Censo 2000* [online]. Available from: http://www.ibge.gov.br/ [Accessed 4 May 2009].

Le Breton, D., 2006. *Sociologia do corpo* [Sociology of the body]. Petrópolis: Vozes.

Okie, S., 2006. Fighting HIV: lessons from Brazil. *New England Journal of Medicine*, 354 (19), 1977–1981.

Parker, R., 2003. Building the foundations for the response to HIV/AIDS in Brazil: the development of HIV/AIDS policy. *Divulgação em Saúde para Debate*, 27, 143–183.

Parker, R. and Aggleton, P., 2003. HIV and AIDS-related stigma and discrimination: a conceptual framework and implications for action. *Social Science & Medicine*, 57 (1), 13–24.

Pierucci, A.F. and Prandi, R., 2000. Religious diversity in Brazil: numbers and perspectives in a sociological evaluation. *International Review of Sociology*, 15 (4), 629–639.

Prandi, R., 1991. *Os candomblés de São Paulo* [Candomblé in São Paulo]. São Paulo: HUCITEC-EDUSP.

Prandi, R., 2001a. *Encantaria Brasileira* [Brazilian enchantment]. Rio de Janeiro: Pallas.

Prandi, R., 2001b. *Mitologia dos orixás* [Mythology of the *orixás*]. São Paulo: Companhia das Letras.

Prandi, R., 2004. O Brasil com axé: candomblé e umbanda no mercado religioso [Brazil and *axé*: Candomblé and Umbanda in the religious market]. *Estudos Avançados*, 18 (52), 223–238.

Revista Atotô Programa Estadual de DST/AIDS de Pernambuco, 2001. Revista Atotô: Cartilha de prevenção as DST/AIDS Dirigida aos Participantes dos cultos Afro-Brasileiros [Prevention pamphlet for STD/AIDS tailored towards participants of Afro-Brazilian religions]. Recife: Programa Estadual de DST/AIDS [State STD/AIDS Program].

Rios, L.F., 2000. A fluxização da umbanda carioca e do candomblé baiano em Terras Brasilis e a reconfiguração dos campos afro-religiosos locais [The fluctuation of *Umbanda* from Rio de Janeiro and *Candomblé* from Bahia in Brazilian terrain and the reconfiguration of local Afro-religions]. *Ciudad Virtual de Antropología y Arqueología. Congreso Virtual 2000.* Available from: http://www.naya.org.ar/congreso2000/ponencias/Luis_Rios.htm [Accessed 9 November 2002].

Rios, L.F., 2004. *O feitiço do Exu-um estudo comparativo sobre parcerias e práticas homossexuais entre homens jovens candomblesistas e/ou integrantes da comunidade entendida do Rio de Janeiro* [The enchantment of Exu: a comparative study of homosexual partnerships and practices of young male practitioners of *Candomblé* and/or linked to the gay community in Rio de Janeiro]. Doctorate thesis. Universidade do Estado do Rio de Janeiro.

Rios, L.F., Paiva, V., Maksud, I., Oliveira, C., Cruz, C., Silva, C., Terto, V., Jr., and Parker, R., 2008. Os cuidados com a "carne" na socialização sexual dos jovens [The vigilance of the flesh in the sexual socialization of youth]. *Psicologia em Estudo*, 13 (4), 673–682.

Sahlins, M., 1985. *Islands of history*. Chicago: University of Chicago Press.

Sahlins, M., 2000. *Culture in practice: selected essays*. New York: Zone Press.

Segato, R., 1995. *Santos e daimones* [Saints and demons]. Brasília: UNB.

Silva, V., 1994. *Candomblé e umbanda: caminhos da devoção brasileira* [Candomblé and Umbanda: paths of Brazilian devotion]. São Paulo: Ática.

Vogel, A., Mello, J.E., and Barros, J., 1993. *A galinha d''angola, iniciação e identidade cultural afro-brasileira* [The Angolan chicken, initiation and the cultural identity of Afro-Brazilians]. Rio de Janeiro: Pallas/EDUFF.

A time for dogma, a time for the Bible, a time for condoms: Building a Catholic theology of prevention in the face of public health policies at Casa Fonte Colombo in Porto Alegre, Brazil

Fernando Seffner[a], Jonathan Garcia[b], Miguel Muñoz-Laboy[c] and Richard Parker[c,d]

[a]Education Department, Federal University of Rio Grande do Sul, Porto Alegre, Brazil; [b]Center for Interdisciplinary Research on AIDS, Yale School of Public Health, Yale University, New Haven, CT, USA; [c]Department of Sociomedical Sciences, Mailman School of Public Health, Columbia University, New York, NY, USA; [d]ABIA, Rio de Janeiro, Brazil

The Casa Fonte Colombo (CFC) is a religious organisation that assists people living with HIV/AIDS (PLWHA). The funding for its activities comes from public sources such as the Brazilian National STD/AIDS Program as well as the Catholic Church. Capuchin (Franciscan) priests run the CFC and it has an extensive group of volunteers made up mostly of women. Between 2006 and 2009, we observed daily life at the CFC and interviewed priests, volunteers, employees, service providers, and clients. We also attended meetings, group sessions, and celebrations. Everyday actions carried out by the CFC reveal the efforts to resolve the tension between the position of the Catholic Church and the Brazilian state in the politics of AIDS. These efforts affirm that the CFC presents itself as a space where the position of the Catholic Church, as much as the politics of public health, are re-worked, giving way to a progressive act of Catholic prevention and assistance for AIDS that we call 'theology of prevention'.

Introduction

Thinking about prevention of AIDS in theological terms

The sometimes tumultuous relationship between the Catholic Church and the Brazilian National STD/AIDS Program[1] is well known amongst Brazilians. There has been an abundance of media coverage over the years. These include public declarations, official statements, opinion pieces, television debates, and interviews detailing papal pronouncements. Officially, the rhetoric used by the Church justifies their opposition based on insufficient effectiveness ('condoms do not block the virus'). Other times they use arguments that question the moral order ('using condoms goes against the moral teachings of the church'). Periodically there is a mixture of both motives evident in the same statement:

In addition to condoms not being 100% effective, condoning their use would invite behaviour that is incompatible with human dignity ... The use of condoms ends up stimulating, even if it we don't intend it to, unrestrained sexual practices ... Condoms offer a false sense of security and they don't preserve the fundamental. (Silberstein 2008, p. 57)

Critiques of the Brazilian Catholic Church's position in relation to the use of condoms as a factor in the prevention of HIV often invoke the phrase, 'The Catholic Church is out of date'. This is a common belief so often repeated in one of its numerous variants including: the Church says one thing but followers do another, times change but the Church does not, and the Church equates condom use with promiscuous sex. It is worth pointing out that sometimes the discussion is more concentrated on the sensitive subjects associated with AIDS such as male homosexuality, prostitution, and drug use. On the other hand, the Brazilian government can take pride in the Brazilian National STD/AIDS Program whose public health responses are highly regarded in international forums, particularly in the realm of treatment access. The participation of civil society, especially nongovernmental organisations (NGOs), from the very beginning of the Brazilian response to AIDS (Galvão 2000), established a collective public health. The ideologically progressive involvement of human rights-based framings of the right to HIV prevention were developed in the AIDS movement (Parker 2000, Parker and Aggleton 2003).

The Brazilian National STD/AIDS Program and the various state and municipal AIDS programmes have specialised in promoting condom use as synonymous with HIV prevention, which is evident in the AIDS education and prevention materials of the government. The Brazilian National STD/AIDS Program and the public representatives of the Brazilian Catholic church have had a complex relationship for decades about condom use.

We also know the Catholic Church is by no means monolithic and there is some room for negotiation at the grassroots (Murray *et al.* 2011). There is a growing collaboration among the government and religious groups partly as a result of the accomplishments of the Brazilian National STD/AIDS Program (Seffner and Bermúdez 2006), which provides important capital in the negotiations with religious groups (Berkman *et al.* 2005, Seffner *et al.* 2009, Garcia and Parker 2011, Muñoz-Laboy *et al.* 2011, Murray *et al.* 2011).

In writing about the relationship between the Brazilian Catholic Church and the Brazilian government in seeking to respond to AIDS, the Catholic theologian, Father José Antonio Trasferetti (2005) presents the idea of a 'theology of prevention', but does not go into a detailed account of what this concept means in terms of this interception between the principles and pragmatic actions of the Church and Brazilian state. The principles and ideologies of the Church have been used to advocate for a *life of plenty* and AIDS care, especially for children and women, showing a great deal of empathy for people living with HIV and AIDS (PLWHA). On this level the convergence of the Church and the Brazilian state has had some difficulties vis-à-vis condom use, as aforementioned. There is also a pragmatic element of this 'theology of prevention'. Although evangelising is part of the prevention response of the Church, the service orientation of the effort takes predominance in many cases. That is, the activities are not saturated by or preoccupied with the transmission of Church teachings in many cases. The active incorporation of public health principles into a prevention approach has transformed the relationship among churches and health providers. In a sense, the state agencies are seen as partners and not adversaries in the case of the 'theology of prevention'.

This paper has two objectives. The first is to present the findings from a historical ethnography that describes the relationship between the Brazilian state and the Catholic Church in terms of AIDS prevention. To assess the Catholic position, we used as a case study the Casa Fonte Colombo (CFC), based in Porto Alegre, and the STD/AIDS Pastoral, a Catholic national organisation whose headquarters are also located in the same city. The second objective is to unpack the concept of 'a theology of prevention', which will help us to better understand the nature of the processes at work in the interface and collaboration between the State and the Catholic Church for HIV prevention. This article highlights the actions of the CFC and the key figures at the STD/AIDS Pastoral that have become characteristic of and played a fundamental role in the development of a 'theology of prevention' (Trasferetti 2005). Studying the production of a theology of prevention, through the analysis of these two Catholic institutions presents a fruitful strategy to analyse this complex cooperation, which demonstrates positive examples and can garner momentum for future initiatives. The paths that the Brazilian Catholic Church followed in responding to HIV and AIDS are important to examine, especially considering the fact that it participates in various continental networks together with the Brazilian STD/AIDS Pastoral, and it often has a coordinating role that can exert considerable influence on other Catholic religious institutions throughout Latin America.

Methods and context

The research project in Porto Alegre

This study is part of a long-term multisite research project conducted by the Brazilian Interdisciplinary AIDS Association (ABIA) in partnership with the Center for Gender, Sexuality, and Health at the Mailman School of Public Health at Columbia University in New York. After 5 years of conducting interviews and ethnography within religious environments in Porto Alegre, we identified the role of the Catholic response to AIDS in Rio Grande do Sul as a principal focus for further investigation, concentrating on two institutions, the CFC and the STD/AIDS Pastoral, whose national secretariat is lodged in the former organisation and run by the Capuchin Friars (Seffner *et al.* 2009). We used a combination of methodologies, which included archival research, media monitoring, participant observation, key informant and life history interviews, and case studies with the objective of documenting how much importance is attributed to the different religions in relation to the AIDS issue. The Case Fonte Colombo is seen as emblematic of the negotiations between the State and the Church in regards to AIDS in Brazil.

Between 2006 and 2009, we observed daily life at the CFC, and conversed with and interviewed 18 individuals who included Capuchin Friars, volunteers, service providers, and clients. We also attended meetings, group sessions, and moments of celebration.[2] The extended ethnographic observation at the CFC, as well as the study and discussion with researchers from other sites of the larger comparative research project (Recife, São Paolo, Rio de Janeiro, and Brasília) allowed for a complex analysis of many subjects in relation to AIDS and various religious organisations. Among these subjects are the questions of: (1) the relationship between the state and religious institutions in the practice of public politics, (2) a cure (in the specific case of CFC, the pretence of a 'cure' for AIDS does not make up part of its mission, although it does exist in innumerable other situations that involve religious action in the universe of AIDS), (3) the boundaries between treatment and evangelising, and (4) the very definition of what disease is and how a person gets sick. In this text, we trace the history of CFC and its connections with the creation of the STD/AIDS Pastoral and analyse the CFC as a space for negotiating meanings about HIV prevention, and articulating the Catholic Church's doctrine and the existing Brazilian public health guidelines on HIV prevention, all of which produce a new discourse, especially, in the area of prevention.

We assessed the manner in which the responses of the CFC were integrated with the local communities, the broader civil society, specific populations (such as youth), and state agencies (e.g., AIDS programmes at the municipal, state, and federal levels) to impact the broader response to AIDS.

Results

Casa Fonte Colombo: history and operations

The interaction between the directors of the Brazilian AIDS Program and the principle doctrines of the Catholic Church that occurs in the CFC and the STD/AIDS Pastoral does not represent the standard relationship between the State and the Church in Brazil. From the stories of the organisers of the CFC, we gathered that the decision to work with PLWHA was not simple, much less a mere chance, but rather 'a long process of discussion and maturation' between the Capuchins and the Catholic Church. The founders retell the trajectory that led to the founding of the Casa that was inspired by Saint Francis of Assisi, who dedicated his life to caring for the sick. This process began in the end of the decade of the 1990s, when the epidemic had already been present in the country for more than 10 years. The first diagnosed cases appeared in 1983, the same year that the State Health Secretariats in São Paolo and Rio de Janeiro began providing the initial government response to the epidemic. The response from civil society began to surge less than 2 years later with the creation of organisations such as GAPA-SP (the Support Group for AIDS Prevention-São Paulo) and ABIA, the first two nongovernmental AIDS organisations in Brazil (Galvão 2000).

The CFC[3] is a service organisation for PLWHA founded by Capuchin Friars in Rio Grande do Sul, who directly coordinate the diverse services offered to the clients. The Case Fonte Colombo is detached from other AIDS NGOs in the city of Porto Alegre, yet it is a national reference in the field of civil society. Importantly, the national secretariat of the STD/AIDS Pastoral of the Catholic Church is also located in Porto Alegre, which confers a rather significant dimension of influence connecting it to the National Conference of the Bishops of Brazil (CNBB).

The Capuchin Friars are part of the Franciscan movement, seeking to personify the charisma of Saint Francis of Assisi by opting for a simple life and taking care of the sick. Saint Francis of Assisi inspired many religious movements and ways of life, which are not all recognised officially by the Vatican. The Capuchin Reform was recognised by the papacy in 1619 acknowledging the Friars who wanted to live the Holy Gospel of San Francisco: 'to live in poverty, obedience, and chastity'.[4] Life outside of the monasteries is permitted for Friars and they have organised fraternities 'dividing their time between missions, work, and prayer'. The Friars arrived in Brazil in conjunction with Italian colonisation, and their presence in Rio Grande do Sul follows the map of this colonisation, having later expanded to the coastal zones of the state. In this context the CFC is considered a fraternity, and the principal activity of the Friars is to care for the sick outside of hospitals. To be a fraternity means, according to the observations we made in our fieldwork, to have a relationship of humility to other companions that they refer to as a brotherhood.

In re-telling the history of this work, the Friars stress the growing needs related to sickness due to HIV, which were already present within the Catholic Church, and evidenced through concrete cases of HIV-positive priests. Perceiving this need, the first task was to set up a half-way home that offered refuge and boarding to PLWHA, caring for those who had to travel to the capital of the Rio Grande do Sul to undergo medical tests and receive treatment. However, the rollout of medical treatments for HIV in the mid-1990s made it possible for most PLWHA to have access to care in their own regions, and the necessity to travel to the capital diminished. Improved availability of antiretroviral medications promoted an important alteration in the mortality rate so that people were able to live with HIV, long-term. As a result, the Friars modified their project and in 1999 founded the CFC calling it the *Centro de Promoção da Pessoa Soropositiva* (Centre for Promotion of Seropositive People; see Seffner *et al.* 2009).

The Casa is located close to a region of commercial sex work in the city between a commercial zone and an industrial zone. The building, when seen from outside, does not have any identification and could easily pass as a business building. Upon entering the door, visitors encounter an organised space, much like a clinic. After taking a second glance, one would perceive the Catholic symbols, crucifixes/crosses and paintings with religious images, most often of Saint Francis, which are similar to the ones found in many public hospitals in Brazil. The activities offered by the Casa are welcoming and provide assistance for PLWHA, including medical and psychological treatment, spiritual guidance from the Friars, massage therapy, Reiki healing energy sessions, food supplements, clothing donation, professional offices, bathrooms, informative lectures, and referrals to obtain other free services. In general people arrive wanting to know more about the disease and the possibilities of living with HIV.

It is noticeable that the Casa attends to very poor individuals, confirming that the CFC often deals with the demand of the most vulnerable populations. The Casa serves as the national secretariat for the STD/AIDS Pastoral of the Catholic Church, the most important religious branch in Brazil that provides assistance to respond to the epidemic. Another factor that distinguishes the CFC from other AIDS NGOs is its vocation for international cooperation. The Casa participates in and coordinates diverse international networks (in Latin America and also with institutions from other parts of the developing world) that bring together religious initiatives for AIDS. The CFC was also the institution chosen by the Brazilian National STD/AIDS Program to facilitate the technical cooperation with East Timor, which is related to, among other motives, the presence of Capuchin Friars in that country.

Each client can stay one afternoon in the Casa because of space limitations. On this afternoon the person chooses from the activities that are made available by the volunteers and the Friars in which they would like to participate.[5] The Friars coordinate daily life at the House creating a schedule that is delineated by each activity: clothes are distributed at the beginning of the day followed by visits and the daily workshop and at 4:30 everyone gathers in the 'space of conviviality' to pray and go to the dining hall together. The volunteer Friars, usually students from the Franciscan School of Theology, provide services such as Reiki or massage therapy, while others give haircuts or theatrical workshops. The volunteers of the Casa have a variety of specialisations that include doctors, nurses, hairdressers, social workers, psychologists, and professors – every job is important.

This array of services permits the Friars to affirm that the CFC has the legitimacy of 'those that act' in the world of AIDS. The CFC participates in numerous events in the realm of AIDS care, as well as in the form of debates, congresses, journeys, public hearings, media programmes, working groups with the directors of AIDS programmes, among other forums. The Friars indicated that the relationship between the CFC and other AIDS NGOs was initially marked by distrust. Representatives from the Catholic Church, sometimes an adversary of AIDS NGOs, sat down next to those from CFC at forums, as partners in arms, which for many was not licit or even acceptable. The perseverance of the Friars in the execution of service work for AIDS and their continued participation in events began to reduce resistance. According to the evaluation offered by the Friars, there is a difference in language, but not in intention, among the religious discourse and the discourse of other AIDS NGOs. The problem did not seem to be related so much to the form of communication. It had more to do with the Friars being representatives in these 'spaces of AIDS' as well as in the Catholic Church.

The CFC today finds itself well established, as much from a material point of view as from a relational standpoint, with other AIDS NGOs in the city of Porto Alegre and in Brazil. They can claim the same solidarity with governmental agencies commissioned in the public politics of AIDS, especially the Brazilian National STD/ AIDS Program and the Centre for International Technical Cooperation of the Ministry of Health, the bureaucratic body that coordinates the cooperation of Brazil with other countries in the area of AIDS. As the secretariat of the national STD/ AIDS Pastoral, the CFC coordinates AIDS-related activities throughout the country, in parishes, communities, hospitals, other pastorals, precincts, schools and other environments within the Catholic Church. It is interesting also to point out that the CFC is effectively a house, where a community of friars resides in the back section on the second floor (the front is occupied by the STD/AIDS Pastoral and dedicated to providing services to clients). No less than five friars reside and work, study, cook their meals, wash their clothes, occupy themselves with other domestic chores, organise celebrations of faith, and sometimes also receive brothers from other communities as guests.

The category that best defines the CFC is a welcoming refuge of acceptance. While living at the house or during repeated visits, the client is always enveloped in an atmosphere of acceptance from employees, friars, and other clients in modes that are both individual (one-on-one consultations with a psychologist, nurse, physician and so on) and collective (at meals, workshops, or conversations in the courtyard). Because of this, the clients attend the institution regularly, forming new groups of friendship and cohabitation that help them face the situation of living with AIDS. The friars also mobilise the clients to participate in events promoted by the AIDS social movement. For instance, World AIDS day on 1 December, prayer vigils, protests in favour of the Sistema Único de Saúde (the national public healthcare system), and meetings such as the Brazilian AIDS Prevention Congress and the National AIDS NGO meeting. In this way, the CFC also contributes to shaping some of the upcoming leaders in the fight against AIDS, similar to the way other NGOs do.

The negotiation of meanings and the construction of agreements between public health policy and Catholic Church doctrine: a theology of prevention

The relationship between the Catholic Church and the directors of the Brazilian AIDS public health programme have been characterised, in the case of the CFC and the STD/AIDS Pastoral, by an intense negotiation of meanings. This negotiation of meanings and the search for consensus takes place between two doctrines that advocate for PLWHA very differently, but which can nonetheless seek to collaborate. This is the process that we describe as the production of a theology of prevention.

Even though the activities of the CFC are more closely linked to assisting PLWHA, the observation and accompaniment of their activities that we did in this period from 2006 to 2009 suggests that it is possible to think of the institution as a producer of a new culture of AIDS, in particular of the prevention of AIDS. The actions and writings from the CFC produced a multiplicity of meanings about HIV and AIDS, characterised by a pro-positive attitude. The institution addresses issues such as age of sexual initiation, interruption of pregnancy, commercial sex work, conjugal relations between men and women, and the expression of sexual orientation without discrimination. In the CFC, using the terminology 'the client' or the general expression PLWHA, helps to produce a new theology of prevention through situations that encourage reflection. The dialogue between the Friars or the volunteers and the clients is not saturated with the 'transmission of lessons of the Catholic Church', although this dimension may be present at times and in particular aspects. The dialogue with the clients seems to serve more to reflect on issues that revolve around AIDS and that introduce new elements within Catholic thought – hence creating knowledge and affirmations systematised by the Friars in lectures and interviews that expose prevention theology.

The construction of a space, within the structure of the Catholic Church, where AIDS can be a principle focus that is treated with care, seems to be a common desire of both the Church itself and the Brazilian National STD/AIDS Program. After many years of public disagreements between these two agents, a tension that has been well covered by the press, we argue here in favour of the idea that public health officials as much as ecclesiastic leaders made efforts to concretise this space of understanding and action in relation to AIDS, where the observations of the directors of public policy could coexist with respect for the tradition of Catholic doctrine (see also, Murray *et al.* 2011). In this way, the CFC, which was already active in responding to the epidemic for years, was seen as a political partner that was well suited for the health authorities of the Brazilian National STD/AIDS Program as much as it was for the hierarchy of the Catholic Church. We continue to briefly narrate the principle points of this trajectory that allow us to perceive the role of growing importance that the CFC assumes, and in particular the organisation of the Capuchin Friars in the interface between the Brazilian AIDS program (at the national and local levels) and the structure of the Catholic Church.

In a quick summary of the history, the STD/AIDS Pastoral initiated conversations in the second half of 1998 between the Brazilian National STD/AIDS Program of the Ministry of Health and the leadership of the CNBB. After that, experts from the Brazilian STD/AIDS Program collaborated with the Catholic leaders involved in the fight against AIDS to create a rather proactive role that stimulated the creation of this work and dialogue, initially a commission and later as a full Pastoral. On the part of the AIDS Program, we see the financing of trips and meetings of participants in this initial phase. According to information available on the STD/AIDS Pastoral website:

> [...] the Commission organized a meeting for a Solidarity Articulation Workshop, that took place in Brasilia August 1–3, 1999. It was this same commission that organized the first seminar 'AIDS and Challenges for the Church in Brazil', June 12–15, 2000, in Itaici that brought together the Minister of Health José Serra, the Coordinator of national STD/AIDS policy, the Adjunct Coordinator, Raldo Bonifácio Costa Filho, Paulo Teixeira, as well as the president of the Pontifical Council of Health and a representative of the Pope – Javier Barragán, the archbishop emeritus of São Paolo – Cardinal Paulo Evaristo Arns, the representative of CNBB – Dom Eugène Rixen, along with religious figures and leaders of the AIDS movement from all of Brazil, directly or indirectly linked to the Church. http://www.pastoralaids.org.br/index1.php (accessed on 24 June 2008)

The old commission for STD/AIDS of the Pastoral of Health transformed into the Pastoral of STD/AIDS, and in June of 2000 it set up a nationwide structure with regulations, statutes, and rules of procedures and a secretariat with its own coordination and headquarters. Similar to other pastorals, the STD/AIDS Pastoral began creating regional branches following the administrative regions the Catholic Church uses in Brazil, and establishing a presence in dioceses, parishes, and communities. They offered training courses to qualified agents of the Pastoral organised into coordination teams to go out and take action. The installation in dioceses and parishes is always done in consultation and coordination with the bishop or priest. The national structure of the STD/AIDS Pastoral was then entrusted to the Capuchin Friars at the CFC, which were responsible for the National Secretariat of the STD/AIDS Pastoral. This secretariat is the executive head of the Pastoral and the national secretariat is one of the Friars from the CFC.

Official documents of the STD/AIDS Pastoral recognise that members of the Catholic Church have been involved in the response to the AIDS epidemic since the middle of the 1980s, but that continuity of work with HIV and AIDS required closer levels of cooperation between the Catholic Church and the Ministry of Health. In this way, the STD/AIDS Pastoral positioned itself as a partner of the State in the fight against the epidemic. Following the model of other pastorals in the Catholic Church, the STD/AIDS Pastoral defined its mission in accordance with the Church, evangelising men and women. One goal was to work with people with HIV, as well as prevention and advocacy work among Christians. At a second level, they defined themselves as service providers and made reference to this commitment in the expression:

... service for the prevention of HIV and assistance to those who are seropositives: the church assumes this service, and without prejudice, welcomes, harbours, and defends the rights of those that are infected with AIDS. We will also do prevention work, through the awareness of evangelical values, presenting mercy and promoting a better life. (CNBB 2003, p. 22)

Emblematic of theology of prevention, the symbol chosen as the official logo of the STD/AIDS Pastoral is composed of a cross and the traditional red ribbon from the fight against AIDS. According to the official documents:

The logo dynamically unites two symbols of solidarity: the cross and the ribbon. The cross represents the solidarity of God with humanity and through it life triumphs over death. The red ribbon is the symbol of the international fight against AIDS. United, these symbols intend to express the commitment of the church to PLWHA and those that also work to prevent new infections. (STD/AIDS Pastoral 2002)

Another definition that shows up frequently in the official materials we consulted affirms that the work of the STD/AIDS Pastoral can be defined in the following way:

Christians who are capable and committed to the work of prevention and assistance, a Church that is committed to the prevalence of life, according to the teaching of Jesus 'I came so that everyone could have life'. (Seffner *et al.* 2008, p. 166)

Discussion

Arranging converging interests between public health and the Catholic Church involved finding a common partner for the dialogue about AIDS, while avoiding clashes that create greater friction between the two institutions (Murray *et al.* 2011). We show that the CFC played an important role in the creation of this space of dialogue between the public policy related to AIDS and the doctrine of the Catholic Church. We can conjecture that without the existence of the Caphuchin Friars of the CFC and their experience, the creation of the STD/AIDS Pastoral would have encountered many difficulties.

The STD/AIDS Pastoral accomplished, in the wake of what was already done by the CFC, the work of creating spaces within the Catholic Church that were more sensitive and progressive regarding AIDS, as well as addressing other subjects including homosexuality, transgender persons, the age of sexual initiation, drug use, a variety of types of conjugal relations between men and women, different family living arrangements, and particularly the use of condoms as an effective mode to prevent HIV infection. The elaboration of a prevention theology designates a perceptible difference between 'offering' condoms to the clients of CFC and making them 'available' and integrating information about how to prevent HIV and other recommendations where principles and values of Catholicism also enter into play.

Prevention is seen as action that seeks to develop (or revive) in the individual a dimension of humanity and of care, and in this way the use of condoms does not hold the same space that it occupies in the educational materials of the governmental AIDS programmes. But condoms are not missing all together, in so much as they are made available. The Catholic Church does not permit the centrality of condoms, in contrast to campaigns run by public health institutions and AIDS NGOs in Brazil. Instead condoms are always seen in association with other strategies and possibilities. They are not condemned, but they also are not positioned as the only option for prevention. Condoms exist alongside other discourses about prevention. Over several years of observation, upon arriving at the CFC, we encountered a bowl full of condoms, many different brands from all different countries, in a central location in the lounge. This functioned a little bit as decoration, but, more importantly, it was a point of availability of condoms for those who wanted them.

This manner of conceptualising the condom, which is not the 'official approach' of the Church, is useful in serving populations that commonly attend the CFC (such as through events that it promoted) for transgender people, young gay men, commercial sex workers, and drug users. At the meetings that we attended, there were agents of the STD/AIDS Pastoral who were gay but who had found a way to work linked to the Catholic Church, while still manifesting their sexual orientation. In this way, many Catholics view the STD/AIDS Pastoral empathetically by having a more progressive stance, and they perceive the work of the Capuchin Friars as planting the seeds of change. In an articulate and intelligent manner, the STD/AIDS Pastoral has accomplished a growth within the structure of the Catholic Church, utilising two well-defined strategies. The first of these is to approach priests from the most progressive parishes and offer to begin an AIDS programme in their region. The second is to try and contact other Pastorals of the CNBB, such as the Pastoral for the Incarcerated, the Afro-Brazilian Pastoral, the Pastoral for Immigrants, the Pastoral of Land, the University Pastoral, the Pastoral for the Homeless, etc. In this second case, the strategy to establish AIDS as an intersectional topic in the work of other organised pastorals greatly amplifies the radius of action of the STD/AIDS Pastoral and at the same time allows them to establish contact with sympathisers of Liberation Theology or of a more progressive Catholicism.

Another source of growth for the STD/AIDS Pastoral, also modelled after the experience from the CFC, stems from ecumenical dialogues with other religious denominations. It is worth pointing out that, since their beginning, they have hosted some volunteers that are Lutheran and Spiritist. After collaborating in this explicit way they made an effort to include other religious groups, as in the case of planning for the vigil for those who have died of AIDS. The existence of groups that work with AIDS from other religious groups, as well as the annual AIDS-related events, facilitates an interdenominational collaboration around AIDS. In this way, today the STD/AIDS Pastoral is a very ecumenical organisation, welcoming to its team individuals that are Lutheran, Anglican, Spiritist, or from various Afro-Brazilian religions, among others. The STD/AIDS Pastoral, and in particular the CFC, participate today in the leadership of Latin American and global networks that fight against AIDS that are composed by a diverse matrix of religious congregations. The CFC receives delegations from other countries in South America, and frequently runs courses and trainings in other countries and continents, which explains in part why they were chosen by the Brazilian AIDS programme to coordinate Brazil's international cooperation with East Timor.

The case study carried out with the CFC and the STD/AIDS Pastoral demonstrates that HIV and AIDS, aside from creating a source of tension between the State and the Catholic Church, also made possible the emergence of a common ground for dialogue and understanding. These institutions, the older CFC and the newer STD/AIDS Pastoral, are concrete manifestations of this understanding. Today these institutions maintain projects with some funding from the Brazilian National STD/AIDS Program. Through publications and a range of strategic projects, they execute programmes of action that compliment public health policy, in the same way that many secular AIDS NGOs do. At the same time, the fight against AIDS produced an articulation of sectors within the structure of the Church that have more progressive positions on topics like homosexuality, conjugal relations, prostitution, and harm reduction for drug users. Only those that rely solely on what the relatively superficial caricatures sometimes produced by the mass media would think that the State and the Catholic Church have positions that are dramatically in contrast regarding AIDS.

This case study demonstrates that reality is much more complex regarding moments of collaboration and tension with different actors in both fields. It also emphasises the extent to which such processes are historically constructed over time. From a time early in the epidemic when only a few progressive sectors of the Catholic Church clandestinely distributed 'hidden' condoms, we have been able to witness the emergence of a new time when a theology of prevention is actively promoted in conjunction with principles of Catholic doctrine and orientations of public health policy from the Brazilian National STD/AIDS Program. Understanding how such processes of change are gradually constructed over time, through careful dialogue and hard work on the front lines of the fight against HIV and AIDS, can offer key insights into the ways in which we might build more effective responses to the epidemic in the future.

Acknowledgements

This article is based on data collected from the research study titled, Religious Responses to HIV/AIDS in Brazil, a project sponsored by the Eugene Kennedy Shiver US National Institute of Child Health and Human Development (grant number R01 HD050118-05; principal investigator, Richard G. Parker). This national study was conducted in four sites, at the following institutions and by their respective coordinators: Rio de Janeiro (Associação Brasileira Interdisciplinar de AIDS/ABIA – Veriano Terto Jr.), São Paulo (Universidade de São Paulo/USP – Vera Paiva), Porto Alegre (Universidade Federal do Rio Grande do Sul/ UFRGS – Fernando Seffner), and Recife (Universidade Federal de Pernambuco/UFPE – Luís Felipe Rios). Additional information about the project can be obtained via e-mail from religiao@abiaids.org.br or at http:www.abiaids.org.br, the Associação Brasileira Interdiciplinar de AIDS (ABIA) website. Jonathan Garcia was supported by F31 HD055153-02 from the Eugene Kennedy Shiver US National Institute of Child Health and Human Development and by T32 MH020031 from the National Institute of Mental Health. The content of this article is solely the responsibility of the authors and does not necessarily represent the official views of the NICHD, NIMH, or the NIH. We would like to thank Priscila Rodrigues Borges and Luana Rosado Emil from the research project Religious Responses to HIV/AIDS in Brazil team in Porto Alegre, who initiated the relationship with the CFC.

Notes

1. The Brazilian National STD/AIDS Programme has had a number of different names over the course of its history, representing different positions in the institutional and organisational structure of the Ministry of Health. For the sake of simplicity, we will refer to it throughout as the Brazilian national STD/AIDS Program. For more information about the Programme, including its current designation, see the Departamento de DST, AIDS e Hepatites Virais website at www.aids.gov.br.

2. The study was approved by the National Ethics Council of Brazil (CONEP 12352), and it uses clear terms of consent in all information-gathering processes.
3. The identification of the CFC results from an agreement between the researcher and the management of the institution. The final version of this text was read by the Friars who gave their informed consent in their personal names and in the name of the institution and they approved the description of their institution as accurate. The informants are not identified in the text to preserve their anonymity. More information about the CFC can be found at http://www.capuchinhosrs.org.br/fontecolombo.
4. http://www.capuchinhosrs.org.br/ – site of the Order of Capuchin Friars of Rio Grande do Sul.
5. The group of volunteers at the Case Fonte Colombo is mostly made up of women, who stay for years as volunteers. Some of them have worked there regularly since the House opened. This characteristic of stability in the ensemble of volunteers is a difference of the CFC in relation to other AIDS NGOs of Porto Alegre, where the circulation/turnover of volunteers is much greater.

References

Berkman, A., Garcia, J., Muñoz-Laboy, M., Paiva, V., and Parker, R., 2005. A critical analysis of the Brazilian response to HIV/AIDS: lessons learned for controlling and mitigating the epidemic in developing countries. *American Journal of Public Health*, 95 (7), 1162–1172.

CNBB (Conferência Nacional dos Bispos do Brasil), 2003. Diretrizes gerais da ação Evangelizadora da Igreja no Brasil, 2003–2006 [General directives of the Church in Brazil 2003–2006]. Itaici, SP: CNBB.

Galvão, J., 2000. *AIDS no Brasil: Agenda de construção de uma epidemia* [AIDS in Brazil: the construction of an agenda of an epidemic]. São Paulo: Editora, 34.

Garcia, J. and Parker, R., 2011. Resource mobilization for health advocacy: Afro-Brazilian religious organizations and HIV prevention and control. *Social Science and Medicine*, 72 (12), 1930–1938.

Muñoz-Laboy, M.A., Murray, L., Wittlin, N., Garcia, J., Terto, V., Jr., and Parker, R., 2011. Beyond faith-based organizations: using comparative institutional ethnography to understand religious responses to HIV and AIDS in Brazil. *American Journal of Public Health*, 101 (6), 972–978.

Murray, L.R., Garcia, J., Muñoz-Laboy, M., and Parker, R., 2011. Strange bedfellows: the Catholic Church and Brazilian National AIDS Program in the response to HIV/AIDS in Brazil. *Social Science and Medicine*, 72 (6), 945–952.

Parker, R., 2000. *Na contramão da AIDS: Sexualidade, intervenção, política* [The counter indications of AIDS: sexuality, intervention, politics]. Rio de Janeiro: Editora, 34.

Parker, R. and Aggleton, P., 2003. HIV and AIDS-related stigma and discrimination: a conceptual framework and implications for action. *Social Science and Medicine*, 57 (1), 13–24.

Seffner, F. and Bermúdez, X.P.D., 2006. Brazilian leadership in the context of the UNGASS Declaration of Commitment in HIV/AIDS. *Revista de Saúde Pública/Journal of Public Health*, 40 (Suppl. 1), 1–7.

Seffner, F., Gonçalves da Silva, C., Maksud, I., Garcia, J., Rios, F., Nascimento, M., Borges, P., Parker, R., and Terto, V., Jr., 2008. Respostas religiosas à aids no Brasil [Religious responses to AIDS in Brazil]. *Ciencias Sociales y Religión*, 10 (10), 159–180.

Seffner, F., Gonçalves da Silva, C., Maksud, I., Garcia, J., Rios, F., Nascimento, M., Borges, P., Parker, R., and Terto, V., Jr., 2009. Respostas religiosas à aids no Brasil: Impressões de acerca da Pastoral de DST/AIDS da Igreja Católica [Religious responses to AIDS in Brazil: impressions about the AIDS Pastoral of the Catholic Church] *In*: L.F. Duarte, E. Campos Gomes, R.A. Menezes, and M. Natividade, eds., *Valores religiosos e legislação no Brasil: A tramitação de projetos de lei sobre temas morais controversos* [Religious values and Brazilian legislation: legal related to moral controversies]. Rio de Janeiro: Editora Garamond, 155–178.

Silberstein, A., 2008. *Pergunte ao Papa* [Ask the Pope] [online]. São Paulo: Legnar Informática and Editora Ltda. Available from: http://www.reinodavirgem.com.br/doutrinamoral/sintovergonha.html [Accessed 25 April 2008].

STD/AIDS Pastoral, 2002. Bulletin. March. 1(1) [online]. Available from: http://www.pastoralaids.org.br/boletim1.php#3 [Accessed 21 May 2011].

Trasferetti, J., 2005. *CNBB, AIDS e governo: Tarefas para uma teologia da prevenção* [CNBB, AIDS, and government: work toward a theology of prevention]. Campinas: Átomo.

Index

ABC (Abstain, Be Faithful and Condom Use) approach 41, 70, 73

African Independent Churches (AICs) in Mozambique 37, 40–1, 42–4, 44–5

African Methodist Episcopal (AME) churches 104, 106–7, 110–11

African Religious Health Assets Programme (ARHAP) 49, 58, 59

'African Science' concept 15

AIDS, religious enthusiasm and spiritual insecurity in Africa: conclusions 18–19; introduction –miracle cure in Tanzania 6–7; religious enthusiasm - relational realism 7–18

'*Andar fora é manyingui arriscado* ('Fooling around is very risky') 27

anti-retroviral therapy (ART): gender vulnerabilities and home-based care 56–7, 59; pentecostalism and AIDS treatment in Mozambique 37–46; Swaziland 50

akrasia of belief 12

ARV (anti-retroviral medication) 16, 41, 52, 54, 55–6

Assemblies of God (Pentecostal church in Mozambique) 40

axé and response of Afro-Brazilian religion to HIV/AIDS in Recife: Afro–Brazilian religious practices and HIV 134–8; Afro–Brazilian religions 132–3; *axé*, HIV and stigma 140–1; discussion 141–2; introduction 131–2; public health responses 139–40; research settings and methodology 133–4

Baixada Fluminense, Rio de Janeiro 119, 122, 125

'behaviour change' 41

Behrend, H. 17

'belief' concept 11

'beliefs' term 9, 11–14

Black churches in New York City and HIV (Black men who have sex with men): Black churches and community mobilisation 102; community-level responses from Black churches 103–4; conclusions 112–14; findings 105–11; introduction 101–5; methods 104–5; stigma and HIV/AIDS among Black churches 103

Black churches in New York City and HIV (Black men having sex with men) – findings: don't ask, don't tell – private vs. public knowledge 107–9; 'love the sinner, hate the sin' – behaviour vs. identity 105, 106–7; 'your body is a temple,' – physical health and spiritual health 109–13

Black churches in New York City and HIV (Black men who have sex with men) – methods: analytic approach 105; interview and focus groups 104; sample 104

Black men who have sex with men (MSM) 86, 101, 103–5, 109, 111, 112–14

'Born Again' church 16–17, 69. 74

Brazil *see axé*...; Catholic theology...

Brazilian AIDS Prevention Congress 151

Brazilian Interdisciplinary AIDS Association (ABIA) 120, 121, 147, 148

Brazilian National STD/AIDS Program 131, 146, 150, 151–2, 155

Brazilian Research Ethics Commission (CONEP) 134

Bush, George W. 18, 45, 70

Candomblé (religion, Brazil) 133, 134–5

Capuchin Friars (Franciscan movement in Brazil) 148–50, 151–2, 154

Casa Fonte Colombo (CFC), Porte Alegre 145–55

Catholic Church: Brazil 145–55; condom use for disease prevention 78; condoms 151; family planning 71; reproduction within marriage 74

Catholic theology of prevention and public health policies at Casa Fonte Colombo, Porte Alegre, Brazil: discussion 153–5; introduction 145–7; methods and context 147–8; results 148–53

Celestial Church of Christ, Nigeria 76
Centers for Disease Control and Prevention, NYC 113
Changana ethnic group, Mozambique 23–4
Christ Apostolic Church, Nigeria 76
Christian Council of Mozambique (CCM) 40
civic/sanctuary orientation and HIV involvement (Chinese immigrant religious institutions in New York City): description 85; discussion 94–7; HIV 85–6; introduction 84–5; methods 88; results 89–94; social engagement 86–8
civic/sanctuary orientation and HIV involvement (Chinese immigrant religious institutions in New York City) – discussion: institutions comparison 94–6; orientation and HIV involvement 96–7
civic/sanctuary orientation and HIV involvement (Chinese immigrant religious institutions in New York City) – results: Community Welfare Church – civic, Christian 89–90, 95–6, 97; Queens Family church – sanctuary, Christian 90–1; Refuge Buddhist Temple - sanctuary, Buddhist 93–4, 95; Temple of Engaged Buddhism – civic, Buddhist 92–3
Civil Rights Movement 103
Clement of Alexandria 71
Clinton Foundation 41
Commission for Religious Affairs 26
community home-based care (CHBC) 59
community and privately funded rehabilitation centre (Rio de Janeiro) 124–5
community-based organisations (CBOs) 1
Concord Baptist Church, Brooklyn 102
condoms and HIV/AIDS: Catholic Church 151; concept 154; distribution 139; harm-reduction 73–4; Pope Benedict 78; Pope and Christian theology 79; religious institutions 72–3; sex education for the young 71–2; short-term targets 78
conflicts (conservative Christian institutions and secular groups) in SSA – sexualities, reproduction and HIV/AIDS: collaboration 77–9; freedom from stigma/discrimination of sexual orientation and gender 74–7; introduction 66–7; reproductive autonomy 74; sexual and reproductive rights 67–73

Darwin, Charles 18
Davis, Mike 40
don't ask, don't tell (DADT) – private vs. public knowledge 107–9, 111, 112, 114
drug rehabilitation centres (DRCs) 117, 120–1, 128

en/theos (enthusiasm, possessed by a god) term 7
'epistemological double bind' 15
Evangelical Lutheran Church, Tanzania 6
evangelical protestant leaders and institutions, drug use and HIV/AIDS in Rio de Janeiro: discussion and conclusions 127–9; introduction 117–19; methods 119–21; results 122–7
evangelical protestant leaders and institutions, drug use and HIV/AIDS in Rio de Janeiro – methods: data analysis 121; interviewing process and key questions 121; research and social context 119; sample selection and recruitment 120–1
evangelical protestant leaders and institutions, drug use and HIV/AIDS in Rio de Janeiro – results: case studies 124–7; discourses of pastors 122–4

faith-based organisations (FBOs) 1–2, 120, 121, 123, 128
family planning (Catholic Church) 71
focus group discussions (FGDs) in Mozambique 43
Foucault, Michel 134, 138, 141
free love – church-run, home-based carers: conclusions 62; discussion 58–62; introduction 48; methods 51; research setting 49; results 51–8
free love – discussion: HIV/AIDS knowledge – training and empowerment 59–60; leveraging assets – religion and social transformations in care/knowledge 60–2; theoretical framework 58
free love – results: caregiver–client relationship 53–4; care-giving and care of self 58; gender vulnerabilities 56–7; HIV/AIDS care practices 54–6; motivations love and/of knowledge 52; religion and home-based care 57

gender (freedom from stigma/discrimination) 76–7
Global Fund to Fight AIDS, Tuberculosis and Malaria 1, 41
Global Health Council 1–2
Global Public Health (Journal) 2
Grounded Theory 51, 105

harm-reduction 73–4
Health Alliance International (HOI, US) 42
Hepatitis C 94
HIV testing and counselling (HTC) 49
HIV/AIDS care practices: ART treatment 55; disclosure and secondary prevention 56; HIV testing 54–5

HIV/AIDS risk-reduction: church leadership 72; condoms and sex education for the young 71–2; harm-reduction 73–4; religious institutions 72–3; religious opposition to condoms 71
Holy Writ and HIV/AIDS prevention methods 66
home-based care (HBC): Mozambique 40, 42–4; Swaziland 61
homosexuality: API communities 86; Buddhists 97; Black churches 103–114; Christians 69, 97; civic/sanctuary orientation 95; Community Welfare Church, NYC 89; Old Testament 74–5; religious/secular institutions 67; Porte Alegre, Brazil 148, 153, 155; Recife, Brazil 133, 136, 142; Rio de Janeiro, Brazil 121; sub-Saharan Africa 75–6; Temple of Engaged Buddhism, NYC 92
'human rights' and AIDS prevention 77
'human security' term 10
Hume, David 7

Igreja Pentecostal church, Mozambique 43
IMF (International Monetary Fund) 39
Immune system 17
Instituto Brasileira de Geografia Estatística (IBGE) 132
International Conference on Population and Development, 1994 68
International Gay & Lesbian Human Rights Commission 75
International Lesbian, Gay, Bisexual, Trans and Intersex Association 75

Joint United Nations Programme on HIV/ AIDS (UNAIDS) 1, 39, 49, 50, 86
Jurema (religion, Brazil) 133

Kato, David 75
Konda ine (protection from HIV infection) 18

Lamont, J. 67
Last, Murray 12
literature review (religious/secular groups and HIV/AIDS prevention) 67
Loliondo Wonder 6–7, 8
'love the sinner, hate the sin' (LSHS) – behaviour vs. identity 105, 106–7, 111, 112, 114

Malawi: religious doctrine 76
maUnits (Malawi) see ARV
Ministry of Health (MOH) in Mozambique 40, 42–3
Mock, A. K. 87–8, 89, 91, 97

Mozambique see organisational constraints...; Pentecostalism and AIDS treatment...
'mugagira' tree 16
Mwasapila, Anbilikile 6–7, 7–8

National AIDS Programme see Brazilian National AIDS Programme
National Conference of the Bishops of Brazil (CNBB) 148, 152, 154
National Emergency Response Council on HIV/AIDS (NERCHA) 49, 50
National Health HIV/AIDS Strategy 103
National Health System, Mozambique 41
National Secretariat against Drugs (SENAD) in Brazil 118
National Week of Prayer for the Healing of AIDS 104
New Testament: dignity of every person 74; extra-marital sex 69; literature review 67; marriage 68
New York City Department of Health and Mental Hygiene (NYCDOHMH) 86, 103
New York City (NYC) see Black churches...; civic/sanctuary orientation
Nicene Creed 12
non-governmental organisations (NGOs): social inequality/religious culture and HIV 2
non-governmental organisations (NGOs, Mozambique): AICs 40, 42; AIDS funding 40; Christian churches 40; community-based assistance and care 32; Health Alliance International 42; management 32
non-governmental organisations (NGOs, Porto Alegre, Brazil): AIDS 146, 148–51, 153, 155
non-governmental organisations (NGOs, Rio de Janeiro, Brazil): AIDS-related 120; church and leadership/network 125; condom use 126; Evangelical AIDS 122
NYC see New York City

Old Testament: condom use 70–1; homosexuality 74–5; literature review 67
Organisation of Mozambican Women (OMM) 45
Organisation of Zionist Pentecostal Churches ('OISPM') in Mozambique 26
organisational constraints in religious involvement with HIV/AIDS (Mozambique): background 22–3; conclusions 33–4; data and method 23–4; organisational dynamics of religious marketplace 24–6; religious organisations in HIV prevention 26–31; religious organisations and HIV/AIDS-related assistance 31–2

Pai Claudio 137–9
Pai Fernando 138
Pai João 135–8, 140
'*Pensa direito, usa Jeito*' ('Think straight, use condom') 27
Pentecostal Church, Kampala, Uganda 69–70
Pentecostal (Zionist) churches in Mozambique 25–6, 37–44
Pentecostalism: Africa 15; idol worship 17; spiritual insecurity 17
Pentecostalism and AIDS treatment in Mozambique – HIV prevention through anti-retroviral therapy: ART scale-up – treatment and prevention 41–2; churches and ART scale-up in two provinces 42–4; conclusions – services and religious communities 44–6; inequality, HIV and church growth 39–41; introduction 37–8
People Living with HIV (PLHIV) 131, 132, 139–40, 141
People Living with HIV/AIDS (PLWHA) 49, 50, 72, 146, 148–9, 151
Pew Forum, US 7, 101
Piot, Peter 39
'politics of personhood' 18
Pope Benedict XVI: condoms 72–3, 78
Presidential Advice Commission on HIV/AIDS (PACHA, US) 102
President's Emergency Plan for AIDS Relief (PEPFAR, US) 1, 41
prevention of maternal to child transmission (pMTCT) in Mozambique 42
programmatic vulnerability in Brazil 118
prostituição (prostitution) in Mozambique 39, 41
Protestant church, Mozambique 29

quilombos in Brazil 132

Reino de Deus (Pentecostal church in Mozambique) 40
religious enthusiasm – relational realism in Tanzania: description 7–10; framework 14–18; spiritual insecurity 10–11; what's wrong with talking about beliefs? 11–14
religious health assets (RHAs) 49, 58, 60, 62
religious institutions in NYC: activist 87; civic 87; evangelical 87; social engagement: sanctuary 87
religious opposition to condoms 71
religious organisations (ROs) in Mozambique 22–6, 28, 31–2, 33–4
research setting (free love): Kingdom of Swaziland 50; Shiselwani Reformed Church home-based care organisations 50–1, 52

Rural Income Survey, 2008 in Mozambique 39

same-sex partnerships in sub-Saharan Africa 75
Satan and God 17, 30
Seventh Day Adventist Church, Zimbabwe 71–2
sex and the *terreiros* (Recife, Brazil) 136–8
sexual orientation (freedom from stigma/discrimination) 74–6
sexual and reproductive rights (Conservative Christian institutions and secular groups): HIV/AIDS risk-reduction 70–4; sexual autonomy 68–70
Shiselwani Reformed Church home-based care organisations (SRC-HBC) 50–1, 52, 57, 59, 60–1
Sistema Único de Saúde (national public healthcare system) in Brazil 151
Smith, S. M. 78
South African Catholic Bishop's Conference 73
state-funded rehabilitation centre (Rio de Janeiro) 125–8
STD/AIDS Pastoral, Brazil 147, 148–9, 152, 153–4
structural adjustment programme (SAP) in Mozambique 39
sub-Saharan Africa (SSA): homosexuality 75–6; religious health assets 59; religious laws 75; same-sex partnerships 75; sex with non-spouse/cohabiting partner 69; *see also* conflicts…
Swaziland 49–50, 58, 61–2
'system of belief' 13

Tanzania *see* religious enthusiasm…
terreiros (temples) in Recife 133–42
'theology of prevention' in Brazil 147
Tilly, Charles 9
Townsend, Chris 73
Trasferretti, Antonio 146
'typical churches' in mid–western USA 87

Umbanda (religion, Brazil) 133
UNAIDS *see* Joint United Nations Programme on HIV/AIDS
United Nations Development Programs (UNDPs) 10
United Nations Population Fund (UNFPA) 1
United States (US): sexual abstinence 61–2

Vatican, the 27, 73, 149
voluntary counselling and testing (VCT) 56, 59

Western Christendom 13
Winfield, N. 78
witches in Soweto 14–15
World Bank 39, 41
World Health Organization (WHO) 1, 68, 118

Xangô (religion, Brazil) 133, 134, 135
xitique (individual resource-pooling) in Mozambique 26

'your body is a temple' (YBIT) – physical health and spiritual health 109–11, 113–14

Zion Christian Church (ZCC) in Mozambique 43